# MATERNITY

---

## FIRST-TIME MOM'S GUIDE

---

*Essential Pregnancy Tips and Worldwide Best Practices for a Healthy Journey*

By Kayren K. Mariirk

TABLE OF CONTENT

# INTRODUCTION

As I sat in the dimly lit nursery, running my fingers over the tiny onesies and imagining the pitter-patter of little feet, a wave of excitement washed over me. I was expecting my first child, and with each passing day, the anticipation and wonder of motherhood grew stronger within me.

During those early months of pregnancy, I found myself immersed in a whirlwind of emotions, questions, and uncertainties. From the thrill of seeing those two pink lines on the pregnancy test to the awe-inspiring moments spent listening to the rhythmic thump of my baby's heartbeat, The sheer magnitude of what awaited me was overwhelming.
Amidst the joy and excitement, however, I couldn't shake the nagging feeling of apprehension. As a first-time mom-to-be, I was flooded with a myriad of questions and concerns. What should I eat? How much exercise is safe? What should I expect during labor and delivery? The plethora of pregnancy books lining the shelves of bookstores offered some guidance, but I found myself craving a resource that spoke directly to me—a modern, comprehensive guide tailored specifically for first-time moms like myself.

It was during one particularly sleepless night, as I tossed and turned, my mind buzzing with thoughts of cribs and car seats, that the idea for this book began to take shape. Drawing from my own experiences, as well as insights gleaned from fellow moms, healthcare professionals, and experts in the field, I envisioned a book that would serve as a trusted companion and confidante for first-time moms embarking on their own journey into motherhood.

With pen in hand and heart aflame with passion, I set out to create a resource that would not only provide practical advice and guidance but also offer reassurance, inspiration, and a sense of camaraderie to women navigating the joys and challenges of pregnancy for the first time.

And so, fueled by a desire to empower and uplift my fellow mothers-to-be, I poured my soul into this book, sharing my own triumphs and tribulations, as well as the wisdom and insights I had gathered along the way. It is my hope that within these pages, new moms will find solace, support, and the courage to embrace the extraordinary journey of pregnancy with grace, confidence, and boundless love.

For me, writing this book has been more than just a labor of love—it has been a testament to the transformative power of motherhood and the unbreakable bond that connects us all as mothers, daughters, and sisters on this incredible journey called life.

Dear Expectant Mother,

As you embark on this extraordinary journey of pregnancy and motherhood, I want to remind you of the incredible strength, resilience, and support that resides within you. You are capable of more than you know, and you have everything you need to thrive during pregnancy and beyond.

There will be moments of uncertainty, moments of doubt, and moments when the weight of responsibility feels overwhelming. But in those moments, I want you to remember this: you are not alone. You are surrounded by a community of mothers, sisters, and friends who stand ready to offer their support, guidance, and love whenever you need it.

You have the strength to overcome any challenge that comes your way, the resilience to bounce back from setbacks, and the courage to face the unknown with grace and determination. Trust in yourself, trust in your body, and trust in the incredible journey of motherhood that lies ahead.

And remember, it's okay to ask for help. Seeking support from healthcare providers, loved ones, and fellow mothers is a sign of strength, not weakness. Lean on your support network, share your fears and joys, and know that together, we are stronger.

As you navigate the ups and downs of pregnancy and motherhood, hold onto the knowledge that you are capable, you are worthy, and you are loved. You've got this, mama. And I am cheering you on every step of the way.

With love and admiration,
Kayren K. Mariirk

# Chapter 1

# Preparing for Pregnancy

Preparing for pregnancy is an exciting and important step on your journey to motherhood. It's a time to not only ensure your body is ready to support a growing baby but also to optimize your overall health and well-being.

Before conception, it's essential to focus on preconception health. This involves adopting healthy lifestyle habits such as eating a balanced diet rich in nutrients, maintaining a healthy weight, and avoiding harmful substances like tobacco and excessive alcohol. Taking prenatal vitamins containing folic acid is also recommended to support the healthy development of your baby's neural tube.

In addition to physical health, preparing for pregnancy also involves addressing emotional and mental well-being. Managing stress, practicing relaxation techniques, and fostering open communication with your partner are important aspects of preparing for the emotional journey of pregnancy.

Furthermore, it's crucial to consult with your healthcare provider before attempting to conceive. They can offer personalized advice based on your medical history and help identify any potential risk factors that may need to be addressed before pregnancy.

Preparing for pregnancy is a holistic endeavor that encompasses physical, emotional, and mental aspects of health. By taking proactive steps to optimize your well-being before conception, you can lay a strong foundation for a healthy and fulfilling pregnancy journey.

# Preconception Health

Prioritizing preconception health is essential for laying the foundation for a healthy pregnancy. Let's look at each of those aspects more closely:

1. **Healthy Diet:** Before trying to conceive, I made a conscious effort to improve my diet, focusing on nutrient-rich foods like fruits, vegetables, whole grains, and lean proteins. Incorporating these foods into my meals not only helped me maintain a healthy weight but also provided essential nutrients for fertility and fetal development.

2. **Maintaining a Healthy Weight:** Like many women, I struggled with maintaining a

healthy weight before pregnancy. However, I knew that achieving a healthy weight was crucial for optimizing my fertility and reducing the risk of complications during pregnancy. With guidance from a healthcare provider, I embarked on a journey to prioritize nutritious eating and regular exercise, ultimately achieving a weight that felt right for me and my future baby.

3. **Regular Exercise:** Exercise has always been an important part of my life, but I knew that maintaining a regular exercise routine before pregnancy was especially important. Not only did exercise help me manage stress and maintain a healthy weight, but it also improved myoverall well-being and prepared my body for the physical demands of pregnancy and childbirth.

4. **Avoiding Harmful Substances:** Limiting or avoiding alcohol, tobacco, and illicit drugs before conception is important for optimizing fertility and reducing the risk of birth defects

5. **Managing Chronic Conditions:** Managing chronic health conditions before pregnancy can improve outcomes for both mother and baby.Remember that every woman's experience with managing chronic health conditions in preparation for pregnancy is unique. It is essential to work closely with

your healthcare team to develop a personalized care plan that meets your individual needs and ensures the best possible outcomes as you prepare to conceive a baby.

6. **Taking Prenatal Vitamins:** One of the first steps I took in preparing for pregnancy was to start taking prenatal vitamins containing folic acid. I knew that folic acid was crucial for preventing neural tube defects, so I made it a priority to start supplementation before conception.

# Fertility Awareness

Understanding fertility and menstrual cycles can help women identify their most fertile days and optimize their chances of conception. Let us take a closer look at each of these aspects:

**Tracking Menstrual Cycles:** We all know that menstrual cycle is the monthly series of changes a woman's body goes through in preparation for pregnancy.
On average, a menstrual cycle lasts about 28 days, although cycles can vary in length from woman to woman and even from month to month.
To track menstrual bleeding start by tracking the start date of your period each month. This is usually day one of your menstrual cycle.

Note the duration of your period and any changes in flow or symptoms throughout your cycle.

**Monitoring Cycle Length:**
Before trying to conceive, I began tracking my menstrual cycles using a calendar or a smartphone app, keeping track of the length of my cycles and the timing of ovulation, I was able to identify my most fertile days and maximize my chances of conception.

The basic way to track the length of your menstrual cycle is by counting the number of days from the first day of your period to the day before your next period starts.

Record this information on a calendar, in a journal, or using a menstrual cycle tracking app which is usually automated and very easy to use.

**Observing Changes in Cervical Mucus:**
Cervical mucus is a natural fluid produced by a woman's body in her cervix, which is the lower part of the uterus. Think of it like a helpful guide for sperm on their journey to meet an egg.

The amount and texture of cervical mucus change throughout your menstrual cycle. Around ovulation, it becomes clear, stretchy, and slippery, like raw egg whites. This is a sign that you're most fertile and ready to conceive.

You can check your cervical mucus by simply wiping with clean toilet paper or your fingers. Pay attention to its color, consistency, and feel.

By tracking changes in cervical mucus, you can predict when you're most likely to ovulate and plan intercourse for the best chance of getting pregnant.

**Monitoring Basal Body Temperature:** Basal body temperature (BBT) is your body's temperature when it's at rest, like when you wake up in the morning before you do anything else. It's your lowest body temperature during a 24-hour period.
BBT is like using your body as a thermometer to measure subtle changes in temperature, By taking your temperature at the same time every morning (best time is few minutes after you wake up) and recording it on a chart or app, you can see patterns in your BBT throughout your menstrual cycle.
Before ovulation, your BBT tends to be lower. After ovulation, it usually rises slightly and stays higher until your next period. This rise in temperature can help you know when you've ovulated.
Tracking your BBT can help you figure out when you're most fertile and when the best time is to try to conceive if you're planning to have a baby.
So, think of BBT as your body's way of telling you what's going on inside, especially when it comes to ovulation and fertility.

**Using Ovulation Predictor Kits:** Ovulation predictor kits (OPKs) are like little tools that help you figure out when you're about to ovulate. They work by detecting changes in your body's hormones, specifically a hormone called luteinizing hormone (LH), which surges just before ovulation.

You use an OPK by peeing on a stick or dipping it into a cup of urine. Most kits come with instructions on when and how often to test, usually starting a few days before you expect to ovulate.

After you've done the test, you'll see lines or symbols on the stick. If the test line is as dark as or darker than the control line, it means you're about to ovulate.

Once you get a positive result, it means ovulation is likely to happen in the next 24-36 hours. It's time to get busy if you're trying to conceive! Personally Ovulation predictor kits (OPKs)became my go-to tool for pinpointing ovulation and identifying my most fertile days.

**How to use ovulation predictor kits**

Using ovulation predictor kits (OPKs) is a straightforward process that can help you identify your most fertile days when trying to conceive. Here's a step-by-step guide on how to use OPKs effectively:

*Choose the Right Kit:*
There are various brands of OPKs available, including strips, midstream tests, and digital tests. Choose the type that you find most convenient and easy to use.

*Start Testing at the Right Time:*
Begin testing several days before you expect to ovulate, typically around mid-cycle for women with

regular 28-day cycles. Adjust the start date based on the length of your menstrual cycle.

*Understand How to Collect Urine:*
Follow the instructions provided with the OPK kit carefully. Most kits require you to collect a urine sample in a clean container or use the test directly in your urine stream.

*Perform the Test:*
Open the OPK kit and remove the test strip or midstream test. Hold it by the handle or grip end to avoid touching the testing area.
Dip the test strip into the urine sample or hold the absorbent tip of the midstream test in your urine stream for the specified amount of time, usually a few seconds.

*Read the Results:*
After the specified testing time (usually a few minutes), read the results according to the instructions provided with the kit.
Most OPKs will display two lines: a control line and a test line. When the test line is the same shade or darker than the control line, the test is considered successful.
Some digital OPKs provide a smiley face or other symbol to indicate a positive result.

*Interpret the Results:*
A positive result indicates that your LH surge has been detected, and ovulation is likely to occur within the next 24-36 hours.
Plan to have intercourse within this fertile window to maximize your chances of conception.

Continue Testing Daily:
Continue testing with the OPK daily until you receive a positive result or until your cycle endsSome women may experience more than one LH surge in a single cycle, so it's essential to continue testing until ovulation is confirmed.

Chart and Record the Results:
Keep track of your OPK results on a calendar, in a journal, or using a fertility tracking app.
Record the date, time, and result of each test to identify patterns in your LH surge and predict ovulation in future cycles.
By following these steps and consistently using OPKs, you can accurately identify your fertile days and optimize the timing of intercourse when trying to conceive. If you have questions or concerns about using OPKs or your fertility, consult with a healthcare provider for personalized guidance and support.

# Essential Steps Before Conception

Taking certain steps before conception can help prepare both the body and mind for pregnancy. Here's a more detailed look at each aspect:

**Consulting with Healthcare Providers:** Before trying to conceive, I scheduled a preconception check-up with my healthcare provider. During this visit, we discussed my medical history, reviewed any medications I was taking, and addressed any concerns or questions I had about pregnancy and childbirth.

**Addressing Medical Conditions:** To manage a chronic health condition before pregnancy, make sure to consult professional healthcare providers for personalized advice. Adjust medications as adviced by your health care providers for safety. Also ensure optimal disease control through regular monitoring and lifestyle modifications. Adopt a balanced diet, regular exercise, and stress management. In addition, consider genetic counseling for hereditary conditions. Seek emotional help to deal with the difficulties. Collaborate closely with healthcare providers to develop a tailored plan for a healthy pregnancy.

**Reviewing Medications**: Before trying to conceive, I reviewed my medications with my healthcare provider to ensure they were safe to continue during pregnancy. In some cases, adjustments were made to my medications to minimize any potential risks to the baby.

**Avoiding Harmful Exposures:** Minimizing exposure to harmful substances was another important step I took before conception. I made it a priority to avoid environmental toxins, radiation, and certain medications that could pose a risk to the baby's health.

**Preparing Emotionally and Mentally:** Finally, I took time to prepare emotionally and mentally for pregnancy and parenthood. I talked openly with my partner about our hopes, fears, and expectations for the journey ahead, and we made plans to support each other every step of the way.

By focusing on preconception health, fertility awareness, and essential steps before conception, I felt confident and empowered as I embarked on the journey of pregnancy and motherhood.

# Planning for Parenthood: A First-Time Mother's Guide

Preparing for parenthood as a first-time pregnant woman is an exciting yet sometimes daunting task. It involves careful consideration and thoughtful planning to ensure a smooth transition into this new phase of life.

Begin by taking stock of your current lifestyle and envisioning how it will evolve once your baby arrives. Consider practical aspects such as living arrangements, childcare options, and financial preparation. Creating a budget and establishing a savings plan can help alleviate stress and ensure you're financially prepared for the expenses that come with parenthood.In addition to logistical planning, it's essential to cultivate a supportive network of friends, family, and healthcare providers who can offer guidance and encouragement along the way. Seek out parenting resources, such as books, classes, and support groups, to enhance your knowledge and confidence as you prepare for the joys and challenges of parenthood.

Furthermore, take time to nurture your relationship with your partner and communicate openly about your hopes, fears, and expectations for the journey ahead. Parenthood is a shared experience, and fostering a strong foundation of love and support within your relationship will be invaluable as you navigate the joys and complexities of raising a child together.

Remember, planning for parenthood is an ongoing process that evolves as your pregnancy progresses and your baby grows. Embrace the journey with an open heart and a spirit of curiosity, knowing that each step you take brings you closer to the incredible gift of becoming a parent.

# Chapter 2

# First trimester : week 1-12

## Confirming Pregnant

Confirming pregnancy marks the beginning of an extraordinary journey into motherhood, filled with anticipation, excitement, and a touch of apprehension. As a first-time mom, the process of confirming pregnancy unfolded as a series of profound moments, each imbued with its own significance and emotion

As for me confirming pregnancy was an extraordinary moment, etched vividly in my memory as a blend of disbelief, exhilaration, and an overwhelming sense of wonder. As a first-time mom, I found myself attuned to the subtlest shifts in my body, keenly aware of the possibility of new life blooming within me. It was during a seemingly ordinary morning that I first sensed something was different. A wave of fatigue washed over me, accompanied by an unexplainable sense of queasiness that lingered throughout the day.

Intrigued by these unfamiliar sensations, I decided to trust my intuition and reach for a home pregnancy test (HPT). With trembling hands, I followed the instructions meticulously, each moment pregnant with anticipation. As the minutes passed, I watched intently as the test developed, heart pounding with nervous anticipation. Then, there it was – two distinct lines, faint yet unmistakable, illuminating the small window with the promise of new life.

Overwhelmed with emotion, I could scarcely believe the reality of what I held in my hands. Tears of joy welled in my eyes as the truth sank in – I was pregnant. It was a moment of profound revelation, a sacred affirmation of the miraculous journey unfolding within me.

With a heart brimming with gratitude and awe, I embarked on the journey of confirming my pregnancy with a healthcare provider. Through the reassuring words of my healthcare provider and the gentle confirmation of a blood test and pelvic examination, the reality of my pregnancy became tangible, anchoring me in the profound significance of this transformative moment.

As I reflect on that extraordinary day, I am reminded of the power of intuition, the beauty of life's unexpected twists, and the profound privilege of nurturing new life within. Confirming pregnancy was not just a milestone; it was a testament to the miracle of creation and the boundless depths of love that awaited me on the journey of motherhood.

In this chapter, we'll explore the various ways to confirm pregnancy, from recognizing early signs and symptoms to using home pregnancy tests (HPTs) and seeking validation from healthcare providers.

**Recognizing Early Signs and Symptoms:**
As a first-time mom, recognizing the early signs and symptoms of pregnancy is an empowering first step on your journey into motherhood. In this section, we'll explore the subtle changes in your body's rhythm that may indicate the presence of new life within you.

*Missed Periods:*
One of the most common signs of pregnancy is a missed menstrual period. If your periods are usually regular and you miss a period, it may be a strong indication of pregnancy.

*Fatigue:*
Feeling unusually tired or fatigued, even if you're getting enough rest, can be an early sign of pregnancy. Hormonal changes and increased metabolic demands may contribute to feelings of fatigue.

*Nausea and Morning Sickness:*
Nausea, often accompanied by vomiting, is a hallmark symptom of early pregnancy, commonly referred to as morning sickness. It can occur at any

time of the day and may vary in severity from woman to woman.

*Breast Changes:*
Your breasts may become tender, swollen, or more sensitive to touch in early pregnancy. Changes in hormone levels can cause these breast changes as your body prepares for breastfeeding.

*Heightened Sense of Smell:*
Many women experience a heightened sense of smell during early pregnancy, with certain odors triggering nausea or aversion. This increased sensitivity to smells is thought to be related to hormonal changes.

*Frequent Urination:*
The need to urinate more frequently than usual, especially during the night, is a common early sign of pregnancy. This is due to hormonal changes and increased blood flow to the pelvic area.

*Emotional Changes:*
Pregnancy hormones can also affect your mood and emotions leading to mood swings, irritability, or heightened emotional sensitivity.

*Cravings and Aversions:*
Some women may experience cravings for specific foods or a sudden aversion to certain smells or tastes. These cravings and aversions can vary widely from woman to woman.

By recognizing these early signs and symptoms of pregnancy, you can begin to listen to your body's cues and prepare for the incredible journey ahead. If you suspect you may be pregnant, consider taking a home pregnancy test or consulting with a healthcare provider for confirmation and guidance.

**Using Home Pregnancy Tests (HPTs):**
Home pregnancy tests (HPTs) offer a convenient and accessible way for first-time moms to confirm pregnancy in the comfort of their own homes. In this section, we'll explore everything you need to know about using HPTs effectively.

*Choosing the Right Test:*
There are various types of HPTs available, including traditional strip tests, midstream tests, and digital tests. Consider factors such as sensitivity, ease of use, and cost when selecting the right test for you.

Timing Your Test:
For most accurate results, it's recommended to take the test in the morning when urine is most concentrated. However, you can take the test at any time of the day, following the instructions provided with the test kit.

*Collecting Urine Sample:*
Follow the instructions provided with the test kit to collect a urine sample. Some tests require you to hold the test strip in your urine stream, while others

may involve dipping the strip into a container of collected urine.

*Interpreting the Results:*
After the specified waiting time, check the test for results. Most tests will display a control line and a test line. A positive result is indicated by the presence of two lines or a symbol indicating pregnancy. A negative result will show only one line or a different symbol.

*Understanding False Results:*
While HPTs are highly accurate when used correctly, false positives or false negatives can occur. Factors such as testing too early, using expired tests, or certain medications may affect the accuracy of the results.

*Seeking Confirmation:*
If you receive a positive result on an HPT, it's recommended to confirm the pregnancy with a healthcare provider through a blood test or pelvic examination. This ensures accurate confirmation and provides an opportunity to discuss prenatal care options.

*Emotional Considerations:*
Taking an HPT can evoke a range of emotions, from excitement and anticipation to anxiety and apprehension. It's important to take care of your emotional well-being during this time and seek support from loved ones if needed.

By understanding how to use HPTs effectively and interpreting the results accurately, first-time moms can confidently take the first step in confirming their pregnancy and embarking on the incredible journey of motherhood.

This stage of confirming your first pregnancy status by using a home pregnancy test (HPT) can be an emotional rollercoaster, filled with anticipation, hope, and apprehension. The moments leading up to checking the test can feel like an eternity, as you grapple with a mix of excitement and nervousness about what the outcome may reveal. It is a profound and deeply personal experience for first-time moms, one filled with hope, anticipation, and an overwhelming sense of wonder at the miracle of new life.

**Seeking Validation from Healthcare Providers:**
After the exhilarating moment of seeing two lines or other positive indicators on a home pregnancy test (HPT), the next step for first-time moms is seeking validation from healthcare providers. This critical stage ensures accuracy, provides guidance, and marks the beginning of comprehensive prenatal care.

Confirming pregnancy through consultations with healthcare providers is a crucial step for first-time moms, providing both reassurance and essential guidance for the journey ahead.

Let's delve into the significance of seeking validation from healthcare providers and the diagnostic tests and examinations used to confirm pregnancy:

**Consultations with Healthcare Providers:**
Consulting with healthcare providers, such as obstetricians, gynecologists, or midwives, offers a comprehensive approach to confirming pregnancy. These professionals are equipped with the knowledge and expertise to provide accurate confirmation and personalized care throughout your pregnancy.

**Diagnostic Tests and Examinations:**
Healthcare providers employ various diagnostic tests and examinations to validate pregnancy and assess its progress:

*Blood Tests:* Blood tests determine the level of human chorionic gonadotropin (hCG), a hormone generated during pregnancy. This test provides a precise indication of pregnancy and can detect it at an early stage.

*Pelvic Examinations:* During a pelvic examination, your healthcare provider assesses the size and position of your uterus, as well as the presence of other physical signs of pregnancy. This examination complements other diagnostic tests and provides valuable information about your reproductive health.

*Ultrasound Scans:* An ultrasound scan uses sound waves to create images of the uterus and fetus. This non-invasive procedure allows healthcare providers to confirm pregnancy, estimate gestational age, and assess fetal development.

**Importance of Validation:**
Seeking validation from healthcare providers offers several benefits:

*Accuracy:* Diagnostic tests and examinations performed by healthcare providers offer a more definitive confirmation of pregnancy compared to home pregnancy tests alone.

*Comprehensive Care:* Confirmation of pregnancy initiates prenatal care, allowing healthcare providers to monitor the progress of your pregnancy, address any potential concerns, and provide essential guidance for a healthy outcome.

*Peace of Mind:* Confirmation from healthcare providers provides peace of mind, alleviating uncertainty and allowing you to focus on preparing for the journey ahead with confidence.

*Empowerment through Knowledge:* By understanding the importance of seeking validation from healthcare providers and participating in diagnostic tests and examinations, first-time moms can take an active role in their pregnancy journey. Armed with accurate information and guidance from healthcare professionals, you can navigate the complexities of pregnancy with confidence and peace of mind.

**Embracing the Reality**

Embracing the reality of pregnancy means acknowledging both the joys and the challenges that lie ahead It means allowing yourself to fully experience the wonder of this incredible journey, even amidst the uncertainties and changes that pregnancy brings.

*Finding Gratitude in Every Moment:*

As you navigate the ups and downs of pregnancy – from the early weeks filled with excitement and anticipation to the later stages marked by physical discomfort and fatigue – I encourage you to find gratitude in every moment. Cherish the flutter of tiny kicks, marvel at the sound of your baby's heartbeat, and revel in the bond that grows stronger with each passing day.

*Navigating the Journey Together:*

Remember, you are not alone on this journey. Whether you find support in loved ones, healthcare providers, or fellow moms-to-be, there is a community of support ready to uplift and encourage you every step of the way.

As you embrace the reality of being pregnant, may you find solace in the knowledge that you are embarking on one of the most beautiful and transformative journeys of your life. Embrace the wonder, embrace the challenges, and above all, embrace the boundless love that awaits you on this extraordinary journey into motherhood.

# Navigating Your Body's Transformations

Pregnancy is a time of profound transformation, both physically and emotionally. From the moment of conception, your body embarks on an incredible journey of growth and adaptation to accommodate the developing life within you.

In the early weeks of pregnancy, hormonal changes may bring about a range of symptoms, from nausea and fatigue to breast tenderness and mood swings. These early signs are often the first indication that your body is undergoing significant changes to support the growth and development of your baby
As your pregnancy progresses, you'll notice more visible changes to your body. Your abdomen will expand as your baby grows, and you may experience discomfort as your ligaments stretch to accommodate your growing uterus. Your breasts may become larger and more tender in preparation for breastfeeding, and you may notice changes in your skin, such as stretch marks and pigmentation.

Throughout your pregnancy, your body will undergo numerous adaptations to support the health and well-being of both you and your baby. From increased blood volume to changes in metabolism and circulation, each transformation is a testament to the remarkable resilience of the human body.

In this chapter, we'll delve deeper into the various ways in which your body changes during pregnancy, offering insight and guidance to help you navigate this transformative journey with confidence and grace.

# First trimester week 1-12

The first trimester of pregnancy, encompassing weeks 1 to 12 after the last menstrual period, is a pivotal time marked by profound biological changes in both the mother's body and the developing embryo/fetus. Here's an in-depth look at the biological processes and accompanying changes that occur during this transformative period:

**Weeks 1-4: Conception and Early Development:**
Week 1 marks the beginning of pregnancy, typically occurring around ovulation when fertilization of the egg by sperm takes place in the fallopian tube.

By the end of week 1 or early week 2, the fertilized egg, now known as a zygote, undergoes rapid cell division as it travels down the fallopian tube toward the uterus.

Around week 3, implantation occurs as the zygote embeds itself into the thickened uterine lining (endometrium). This triggers the release of hormones that support the pregnancy.

By week 4, the embryo begins to form, with the development of the neural tube (which becomes the brain and spinal cord), the primitive heart, blood vessels, and the early structures of the limbs.

**Accompanying Changes and Symptoms:**
Hormonal changes, including a surge in human chorionic gonadotropin (hCG) and progesterone, contribute to common early pregnancy symptoms such as fatigue, breast tenderness, nausea (often referred to as morning sickness), and heightened sense of smell.

Many women may also experience mood swings, increased urinary frequency due to the growing uterus pressing on the bladder, and changes in appetite and food aversions.

**Weeks 5-8: Organogenesis and Growth:**
This period, known as the embryonic stage, is characterized by rapid development and differentiation of major organs and body systems.

By week 5, the embryo's heart begins to beat, and limb buds start to form.

Facial features, including eyes, ears, and mouth, become more distinct.

Weeks 6-7 see the development of essential organs such as the lungs, liver, kidneys, and gastrointestinal tract.

By the eighth week, the embryo has developed into a fetus. It has a recognizable human shape, with distinct facial features and rudimentary limbs.

**Accompanying Changes and Symptoms:**
Nausea and vomiting may peak during these weeks for some women, while others may experience relief from early pregnancy symptoms.
Fatigue and mood swings may persist, and some women may notice changes in their skin, including acne or darkening of the skin around the nipples and abdomen (linea nigra).

**Weeks 9-12: Fetal Growth and Maturation:**
During this phase, the fetus undergoes rapid growth and refinement of its organ systems.
By week 9, the fetus's external genitalia begin to differentiate, and fingers and toes develop.
Weeks 10-12 mark the continued growth and maturation of the fetus, with the development of facial features, fingernails, and hair follicles.
By week 12, the fetus is approximately 2.5 to 3 inches in length and weighs around half an ounce.

**Accompanying Changes and Symptoms:**
Some women may begin to feel the first flutters of fetal movement (quickening) around weeks 11-12, though this can vary widely among individuals.
Breast tenderness and fatigue may lessen for some women as they enter the second trimester, while others may continue to experience these symptoms to varying degrees.

Throughout the first trimester, the placenta develops and becomes the primary source of nourishment and oxygen for the growing fetus.

Hormonal changes continue to play a crucial role in supporting the pregnancy and preparing the mother's body for the demands of gestation.

Overall, the first trimester is a dynamic period characterized by remarkable biological changes and adaptation as both mother and baby prepare for the journey ahead. Regular prenatal care, healthy lifestyle choices, and adequate support are essential for ensuring the health and well-being of both mother and baby during this critical time.

# Navigating Early Pregnancy Symptoms

As you embark on this remarkable adventure, you may find yourself navigating a variety of early pregnancy symptoms that are both new and sometimes challenging to manage. Rest assured, you are not alone. In this guide, we'll explore common early pregnancy symptoms and provide tips for navigating them with grace and ease.

1. **Morning Sickness:**
Morning sickness, characterized by nausea and sometimes vomiting, is one of the most well-known early pregnancy symptoms. While it can occur at any time of the day, many women experience it most intensely in the morning. To manage morning sickness, try eating small, frequent meals throughout the day, avoiding strong smells or

triggers, and staying hydrated with ginger tea or lemon water.

### 2. **Fatigue**:

Feeling tired or exhausted is another common symptom of early pregnancy, often attributed to hormonal changes and the body's increased energy demands. Listen to your body and prioritize rest whenever possible. Take short naps, delegate tasks when needed, and try gentle exercise like walking or prenatal yoga to boost energy levels.

### 3. **Breast Tenderness:**

Hormonal variations during early pregnancy can result in breast discomfort or sensitivity. Invest in a supportive bra with good coverage to provide comfort and reduce discomfort You may also find relief from warm compresses or gentle massages to soothe sore breasts.

### 4. **Food Aversions and Cravings:**

Changes in taste and smell can lead to food aversions or cravings during early pregnancy. Listen to your body's cues and honor your cravings when they arise, within reason. Aim for a balanced diet with plenty of fruits, vegetables, lean proteins, and whole grains, while indulging in your cravings in moderation.

### 5. **Mood Swings:**

Fluctuating hormone levels can contribute to mood swings, leaving you feeling elated one moment and tearful the next. Practice self-compassion and be gentle with yourself during this emotional rollercoaster. Engage in activities that bring you joy, whether it's spending time in nature, practicing mindfulness, or connecting with loved ones.

## 6. Increased Urination:

The growing uterus can put pressure on the bladder, leading to increased urinary frequency during early pregnancy. Stay hydrated but consider reducing fluid intake close to bedtime to minimize nighttime trips to the bathroom. Practice pelvic floor exercises to strengthen bladder control muscles and alleviate symptoms.

## 7. Constipation:

Hormonal changes and prenatal vitamins can contribute to constipation during early pregnancy. Increase fiber intake by incorporating more fruits, vegetables, and whole grains into your diet. Stay hydrated, exercise regularly, and consider speaking with your healthcare provider about safe over-the-counter remedies if needed.

## 8. Bloating and Gas:

Hormonal fluctuations and slowed digestion can cause bloating and gas in early pregnancy. Eat smaller, more frequent meals to aid digestion and avoid foods that are known to cause gas, such as beans, cabbage, and carbonated beverages. Gentle exercise like walking can also help alleviate bloating and promote regularity.

Remember, every pregnancy is unique, and your experience of early pregnancy symptoms may differ from others. If you have concerns about the severity or duration of your symptoms, don't hesitate to reach out to your healthcare provider for guidance and support. Trust in your body's incredible ability to nurture and sustain new life, and embrace the journey of pregnancy with grace and resilience.

# Prenatal care Basics

Prenatal care is essential for ensuring the health and well-being of both mother and baby throughout pregnancy. By receiving regular medical check-ups and following recommended guidelines, expectant mothers can minimize the risk of complications and promote optimal fetal development. Here are the key components of prenatal care:

**Early and Regular Check-Ups:**
Schedule your first prenatal appointment as soon as you suspect you're pregnant or have a positive pregnancy test.
During the initial visit, your healthcare provider will conduct a thorough medical history review, physical examination, and possibly a dating ultrasound to confirm the gestational age of the fetus.
Subsequent prenatal visits typically occur once a month during the first two trimesters, every two

weeks during the third trimester, and weekly during the final weeks of pregnancy.

**Medical History and Risk Assessment:**
Your healthcare provider will inquire about your medical history, including any pre-existing health conditions, previous pregnancies, surgeries, and family medical history.
A risk assessment will be conducted to identify any factors that may increase the risk of complications during pregnancy, such as advanced maternal age multiple pregnancies, or chronic medical conditions.

**Nutritional Guidance:**
Proper nutrition is crucial for supporting fetal growth and development, as well as maintaining maternal health.
Your healthcare provider will offer guidance on a balanced diet rich in fruits, vegetables, lean proteins, whole grains, and dairy products.
Prenatal vitamins containing folic acid, iron, calcium, and other essential nutrients may be recommended to ensure adequate nutrition for both mother and baby.

**Screening and Diagnostic Tests:**
Prenatal screening tests, such as blood tests and ultrasound examinations, are used to assess the risk of genetic conditions and birth defects.
Diagnostic tests, such as chorionic villus sampling (CVS) and amniocentesis, may be recommended

for further evaluation if screening tests indicate an increased risk of genetic abnormalities.

**Monitoring Fetal Growth and Well-Being:**
Regular fetal monitoring, including ultrasound examinations and fetal heart rate monitoring, allows healthcare providers to assess fetal growth and well-being throughout pregnancy.
Kick counts, or daily monitoring of fetal movements, may be recommended in later stages of pregnancy to monitor fetal activity.

**Education and Counseling:**
Prenatal care visits provide opportunities for education and counseling on various topics, including childbirth preparation, breastfeeding, newborn care, and postpartum recovery.
Discuss any questions or concerns with your healthcare provider openly to receive personalized guidance and support.

**Emotional Support:**
Pregnancy can be an emotionally challenging time, and prenatal care visits offer opportunities for emotional support and guidance.
Don't hesitate to discuss any fears, anxieties, or mood changes with your healthcare provider, who can offer reassurance and resources for coping strategies.

**Preparation for Labor and Delivery:**
As pregnancy progresses, discussions about birth preferences, labor options, and pain management techniques become increasingly important.
Attend prenatal classes or workshops to learn about the stages of labor, relaxation techniques, and coping strategies for childbirth.

By prioritizing prenatal care and working closely with your healthcare provider, you can optimize your health and the health of your baby throughout pregnancy. Remember that each pregnancy is unique, and individualized care is essential for ensuring a safe and healthy outcome for both mother and baby.

# A Dialogue between Kayren K. Mariirk and Lian(a second time mom)

- Mariirk: Hello Lian
- Lian: Hello Mariirk
- Mariirk: Thank you for agreeing to share your story with the world. It means alot to me.
- Lian: It's with excited that I do this, [laughs] I'm really happy that I can share my story to your readers.
- Mariirk: Can you tell me more about how your first trimester went?

- Lian: Sure. My name is Lian, and I'm now a second-time mom, but let me take you back to my first pregnancy journey. I got pregnant for my first child (daughter) in January of 2018, It was a rollercoaster ride of emotions, uncertainties, and unexpected discoveries. Like many first-time moms, I was filled with a mix of excitement and trepidation as I embarked on this new chapter of my life.
The journey began with the subtlest of signs – a sudden aversion to my morning coffee, an inexplicable fatigue that seemed to settle over me like a heavy blanket. And then, the nausea hit me like a freight train, relentless and unyielding, making even the thought of food unbearable.
As the days turned into weeks, the symptoms only intensified. I found myself battling waves of fatigue that left me struggling to keep my eyes open past midday, and the constant, nagging nausea that seemed to follow me wherever I went.

- Mariirk: That sounds intense. How did you cope with those symptoms?
- Lian: It was tough, especially since I was still trying to wrap my head around the idea of being pregnant. I focused on eating small, frequent meals, sipping ginger tea, and taking naps whenever I could. But amidst the physical discomfort, there were

moments of pure wonder and joy. Feeling those first flutters of movement from within, like tiny butterfly wings brushing against my belly, filled me with an indescribable sense of awe and connection to the life growing inside me.Yet, alongside the wonder, there were also moments of fear and uncertainty.

- Mariirk: Did you experience any specific challenges or concerns during the first trimester?
- Lian: Well! Yes. I experienced sudden onset of cramps and occasional spotting which back then sent me into a panic, fearing the worst with each twinge or ache.
  Navigating the emotional rollercoaster of pregnancy was no easy feat either. Mood swings became a daily occurrence, leaving me feeling like I was riding an emotional rollercoaster with no end in sight.
  [Both laughs]
- Mariirk: It sounds like you went through a lot. How did you navigate those emotional ups and downs?
- Lian: Well, through it all, I found strength in the unwavering support of my partner, family, and friends. Their love and encouragement became my anchor amidst the storm, reminding me that I was not alone in this journey.
- Mariirk: That's great to hear. Did you have any specific questions or concerns about prenatal care during that time?

- Lian: Not really. I was pretty diligent about scheduling my appointments and following my healthcare provider's recommendations. It gave me peace of mind knowing that I was taking proactive steps to ensure a healthy pregnancy.
- Mariirk: It sounds like you were proactive about your prenatal care. Overall, how would you describe your first trimester experience?
- Lian: It was definitely a rollercoaster of emotions and physical changes, but ultimately, it was a beautiful journey of self-discovery and anticipation. Despite the challenges, I wouldn't trade it for anything.
- Mariirk: Thank you so much for sharing your story, Lian. I'm sure it will resonate with many first-time moms who are embarking on their own pregnancy journeys.
- Lian: My pleasure. I hope it helps others feel less alone in the process.

# Questions And Answer Related To The First Trimester

Question 1: How did you manage morning sickness during your first trimester?
Answer: I found that eating small, frequent meals helped alleviate nausea, along with ginger tea and crackers.

Question 2: Were you able to continue exercising during your first trimester? If so, what activities did you find most comfortable?

Answer: I continued with light exercises like walking and prenatal yoga.

Question 3: Did you experience extreme fatigue during your first trimester, and if so, how did you cope with it?

Answer: Yes, fatigue was quite common for me. I tried to rest whenever possible and prioritized sleep at night.

Question 4: How did you handle mood swings and emotional changes during the first trimester?

Answer: I found that talking openly with my partner and practicing relaxation techniques like deep breathing helped me manage my emotions.

Question 5: When did you schedule your first prenatal appointment, and what did it entail?

Answer: I scheduled mine as soon as I found out I was pregnant. The first appointment involved a medical history review, physical exam, and discussion of prenatal care.

Question 6: Were there any foods you avoided during your first trimester, and did you experience any food cravings?

Answer: I avoided raw or undercooked meats and fish high in mercury. Cravings-wise, I couldn't get enough of citrus fruits!

Question 7: Did you encounter any challenges or concerns during your first trimester, and how did you address them?

Answer: I experienced some spotting early on, which was concerning, but it turned out to be relatively normal. I discussed it with my healthcare provider for peace of mind.

Question 8: When did you first start feeling fetal movements during your first pregnancy?

Answer: I started feeling flutters around the second trimester, but it varies for everyone.

Question 9: How did you cope with cramping or discomfort during the first trimester?

Answer: I experienced mild cramping, which I found eased with rest and hydration. If you have any concerns, always consult your doctor.

Question 10: Were there any prenatal vitamins or supplements you took during your first trimester, and did you experience any side effects?

Answer: I took a prenatal vitamin recommended by my doctor, which included folic acid and iron. It didn't cause any issues for me, but everyone reacts differently.

Question 11: How did you manage constipation or other digestive issues during the first trimester?

Answer: I focused on eating high-fiber foods, staying hydrated, and getting regular exercise to help alleviate constipation.

Question 12: Did you experience any changes in your skin or hair during the first trimester, and if so, how did you deal with them?

Answer: I noticed some changes in my skin, like increased oiliness and occasional breakouts. I stuck to a gentle skincare routine and consulted with my healthcare provider for any concerns.

Question 13: Were there any specific prenatal classes or workshops you attended during the first trimester to prepare for childbirth and parenting?

Answer:Yes. I attended prenatal yoga classes and a childbirth education workshop to learn about labor and delivery.

Question 14: How did you manage stress or anxiety during the first trimester, especially with the uncertainties of pregnancy?

Answer: I found relaxation techniques like deep breathing and meditation helpful, along with talking openly with my partner and friends about my feelings.

Question 15: Did you experience any changes in your sex drive or intimacy during the first trimester, and if so, how did you and your partner navigate them?

Answer: My sex drive fluctuated a bit, which is normal during pregnancy. My partner and I communicated openly and found other ways to connect intimately during that time.

Question 16: How did you deal with sleep disturbances or insomnia during the first trimester?

Answer: I struggled with occasional insomnia, but I tried to establish a bedtime routine and create a comfortable sleep environment to improve my sleep quality.

Question 17: Were there any prenatal screenings or tests you opted for during the first trimester, and if so, what was your experience with them?

Answer: I had some routine blood tests and opted for the first-trimester screening for genetic disorders. It was a bit nerve-wracking, but I felt reassured after discussing the results with my healthcare provider.

Question 18: How did you handle work or other responsibilities during the first trimester, especially if you experienced fatigue or other pregnancy symptoms?

Answer: I tried to prioritize self-care and communicate openly with my employer about my needs. Taking breaks when necessary and delegating tasks helped me manage my workload better.

Question 19: Did you encounter any challenges with medication or existing health conditions during the first trimester, and if so, how did you address them?

Answer: I had to adjust some medications with guidance from my healthcare provider to ensure they were safe during pregnancy. It is critical to consult with your doctor.

# Chapter 4

# Second Trimester: Weeks 13-27

During the second trimester of pregnancy, which spans from week 13 to week 27, significant biological, physical, and emotional changes occur as the fetus continues to develop and grow.

Biologically, the second trimester is characterized by rapid growth and development of the fetus. By the end of the first trimester, most of the baby's major organs and structures have formed, and the focus shifts to refinement and maturation. During the second trimester:

**1.Fetal Growth:** The fetus undergoes substantial growth in size and weight. By the end of the second trimester, the baby typically weighs around 2 pounds and measures about 14 inches in length. Organs and systems continue to develop and become more functional.

**2.Organ Development:** While many organs have formed by the end of the first trimester, the second trimester sees further development and refinement of these structures. For example, the brain continues to grow and develop, and neurons begin to form connections. The lungs begin manufacturing surfactant, a chemical required for breathing after birth. The digestive system develops further, and the baby starts swallowing and producing urine.

**3.Skeletal Development:** The baby's bones continue to ossify (harden) during the second trimester. Cartilage is replaced by bone tissue, and bones become stronger and more defined.

**4.Reproductive System:** By mid-pregnancy, the sex of the baby can usually be determined via ultrasound. In male fetuses, the testes begin to descend into the scrotum, while in females, the ovaries continue to develop.

**5.Movement:** Fetal movement, known as "quickening," typically becomes more pronounced during the second trimester. Expectant mothers may start to feel fluttering sensations or gentle kicks as the baby becomes more active.

Physically, the second trimester often brings relief from some of the early pregnancy symptoms experienced during the first trimester, such as nausea and fatigue. However, it also comes with its own set of physical changes:

**6.Visible Baby Bump:** As the uterus expands to accommodate the growing fetus, the baby bump becomes more prominent. Many women start to "show" during the second trimester, and the pregnancy becomes more noticeable to others.

**7.Breast Changes:** The breasts continue to undergo changes, becoming larger and more tender. The nipples may darken in color, and veins may become more visible due to increased blood flow.

**8.Skin Changes:** Hormonal fluctuations may lead to changes in the skin, including pigmentation changes (such as darkening of the nipples and the appearance of a dark line, called linea nigra, on the abdomen), stretch marks, and acne.

**9.Hair and Nail Growth:** Some women experience thicker, shinier hair and faster nail growth during pregnancy due to hormonal changes.

**10.Weight Gain:** Weight gain during the second trimester is normal and expected as the baby grows. On average, women may gain around 1-2 pounds per week during this time.
Emotionally, the second trimester can be a time of increased excitement and anticipation as the pregnancy becomes more tangible. Many expectant parents feel a greater sense of connection to their baby as they begin to feel fetal movements. However, emotional ups and downs are common, and some women may experience anxiety about the upcoming birth or worries about their ability to parent. It's essential for pregnant

individuals to practice self-care, seek support from loved ones, and communicate openly with their healthcare providers about any concerns or emotions they may be experiencing.

# Screening Tests and Ultrasounds

During pregnancy, screening tests and ultrasounds play a crucial role in monitoring the health and development of both the mother and the baby. These non-invasive procedures provide valuable information that helps healthcare providers assess the risk of certain conditions, detect abnormalities, and ensure the well-being of the pregnancy.

Screening tests and ultrasounds provide expectant parents with valuable information about their baby's health and development, empowering them to make informed decisions and receive appropriate care throughout the pregnancy journey. Below is an explanatory list of screening test and ultrasound carried out on pregnant women.

## Screening Tests

**First-Trimester Screening:**
*Nuchal Translucency (NT) Scan:*
**Purpose:** This ultrasound measures the thickness of the fluid buildup at the back of the baby's neck (nuchal fold). Increased thickness may indicate a

higher risk of chromosomal abnormalities, particularly Down syndrome.

**Procedure:** The ultrasound technician will use a transducer to obtain images of the baby's neck area. Measurements are taken, and the results are typically combined with maternal blood test results for a more accurate assessment of risk.

*Combined First-Trimester Screening:*
**Purpose:** Combines the NT scan with maternal blood test results (PAPP-A and hCG) to estimate the risk of chromosomal abnormalities.
**Procedure:** Blood samples are drawn from the mother to measure levels of pregnancy-associated plasma protein-A (PAPP-A) and human chorionic gonadotropin (hCG). Results are then combined with NT scan measurements for risk assessment.
(In other words: You'll have a blood test to check levels of certain proteins, and the results are combined with the NT scan to get a clearer picture of any risks).

**Second-Trimester Screening:**
**Quad Marker Screening (Quadruple Screen):**
**Purpose:** This blood test assesses levels of four substances in the mother's blood to estimate the risk of certain birth defects or chromosomal abnormalities.

**Procedure:** Blood is drawn from the mother to measure levels of alpha-fetoprotein (AFP), hCG, unconjugated estriol, and inhibin A. Results are analyzed to determine the risk of neural tube defects, Down syndrome, and other chromosomal abnormalities. (You'll have a blood test to check levels of different substances, which can give clues about your baby's health).

**Cell-Free Fetal DNA Testing (Non-Invasive Prenatal Testing, NIPT):**
**Purpose:** NIPT analyzes fragments of fetal DNA present in the mother's bloodstream to screen for chromosomal abnormalities with high accuracy.
(In other words, this blood test checks for genetic conditions like Down syndrome with high accuracy).

**Procedure:** A blood sample is drawn from the mother, and fetal DNA fragments are extracted and analyzed. Results provide information about the risk of conditions such as Down syndrome, trisomy 18, and trisomy 13, as well as the baby's sex and certain genetic conditions.
(In other words, a blood sample is taken from your arm, and the lab tests it to look for bits of your baby's DNA).

**Ultrasounds:**

**Dating Ultrasound:**
**Purpose:** Determines the gestational age of the fetus and confirms viability.

(In other words,this ultrasound checks how far along you are in your pregnancy and makes sure everything looks good with your baby).

**Procedure:** A transducer is placed on the mother's abdomen, emitting high-frequency sound waves that create images of the uterus and fetus. Measurements of the crown-rump length are taken to estimate gestational age.

(In other words, a technician uses a small device called a transducer on your belly to take pictures of your uterus and baby)

**Anatomy Ultrasound (Level II Ultrasound):**

**Purpose:** Evaluates the baby's anatomy in detail to detect any structural abnormalities. (In other words,this ultrasound looks at all the details of your baby's body to make sure everything is growing as it should).

**Procedure:** Similar to the dating ultrasound, a transducer is used to obtain images of the baby's body. The technician examines various organs and structures, including the brain, heart, spine, limbs, and internal organs, as well as the placenta, amniotic fluid levels, and umbilical cord position.

(In other words, similar to the dating ultrasound, a transducer is used to take pictures, but this time the technician looks closely at your baby's organs and structures).

**Growth Ultrasounds:**
**Purpose:** Monitors fetal growth and assesses amniotic fluid levels. (In other words, these ultrasounds check how your baby is growing and make sure there's enough fluid around them)
**Procedure:** Similar to other ultrasounds, transducers are used to obtain images of the baby and uterus. Measurements of the baby's head circumference, abdominal circumference, and femur length are taken to assess growth. (In other words, the technician takes measurements of your baby's head, belly, and legs to track their growth over time).

**Specialized Ultrasounds:**
**Doppler Ultrasound:**
**Purpose:** Assesses blood flow through the umbilical cord, placenta, and fetal vessels.
(In other words, this checks the blood flow to your baby to make sure they're getting enough oxygen and nutrients).
**Procedure:** Doppler ultrasound technology is used to measure the speed and direction of blood flow in specific vessels.
(In other words, the technician uses a special type of ultrasound to measure the speed and direction of the blood flow in certain blood vessels).

**Fetal Echocardiography:**
**Purpose:** Evaluates the structure and function of the baby's heart in detail. (In other words, this

ultrasound looks closely at your baby's heart to make sure it's working properly).

**Procedure**: Similar to other ultrasounds, specialized imaging techniques are used to examine the baby's heart chambers, valves, and blood flow patterns (focusing on your baby's heart and how it's beating).

**3D/4D Ultrasound**:
**Purpose**: Provides detailed three-dimensional images of the baby's face and features.

**Procedure**: Specialized transducers are used to capture three-dimensional images of the baby in real-time, allowing for a more lifelike view.
(In other words, the technician uses special equipment to take pictures of your baby from different angles, so you can see them in more details).

Each of these screening tests and ultrasounds plays a crucial role in monitoring the health and development of both the mother and the baby throughout pregnancy. They provide valuable information to healthcare providers, allowing them to identify any potential issues early on and provide appropriate care and support. It's important for pregnant women to discuss the benefits, limitations, and potential risks of these tests with their healthcare provider to make informed decisions about their prenatal care.

# Bonding with Your Baby

As a first-time mom, the journey of bonding with your unborn baby begins long before you hold them in your arms. Understanding the biological processes at play can help deepen your connection and enhance your pregnancy experience.

**Feeling the Love:**
Your body is amazing! It releases a special hormone called oxytocin that makes you feel all warm and fuzzy inside. This hormone helps you feel extra close to your baby, like a super-strong hug from the inside out.

**Baby Talk:**
Guess what? Your baby can hear you! So go ahead and chat with them. Tell them about your day, sing a song, or just say "hello." Even though they're still in your belly, they love hearing your voice.

**Eating for Two:**
Eating healthy isn't just good for you—it's great for your baby too! Foods like fish and nuts have special stuff called omega-3s that help your baby's brain grow big and strong. So munch away,knowing you're giving your baby the best start in life.

**Mindful Moments:**
Take a little time each day to relax and connect with your baby. Close your eyes, take some deep breaths, and imagine all the wonderful things you'll

do together. It's like sending a little love note to your baby!

**Sharing the Joy:**
Don't forget to involve your spouse in the fun! Take them along to your doctor visits, feel your baby's kicks together, and dream about all the adventures you'll have as a family. It's a great way to bond as you get ready to welcome your little one into the world.

**Cherishing Every Moment:**
Bonding with your baby is a journey, and every little moment counts. So savor those kicks, treasure those quiet moments, and know that your love for your baby grows stronger every day.

With each passing day, you're getting closer and closer to meeting your precious little one. So keep smiling, keep loving, and get ready for the incredible adventure ahead!

# Ways a pregnant woman can bond with her unborn child

**Talk to Your Baby:** Your voice is one of the first sounds your baby will recognize. Take time each day to talk to your baby, share your thoughts, dreams, and hopes for the future. You can also read aloud, sing lullabies, or even recite poetry.

**Massage Your Belly:** Gently massaging your belly can help you connect with your baby and promote relaxation for both of you. Use gentle, circular motions and pay attention to how your baby responds to touch.

**Play Music:** Play soothing music or your favorite songs for your baby. Place headphones on your belly and let your baby listen to the melodies. Some studies suggest that babies can recognize music they heard in the womb after birth.

**Practice Mindfulness:** Take moments throughout the day to focus on your baby and your pregnancy experience. Close your eyes, breathe deeply, and visualize your baby's movements. Pay attention to the sensations in your body as you connect with your little one.

**Keep a Pregnancy Journal:** Start a journal to document your pregnancy journey. Write about your thoughts, feelings, and experiences as you prepare to welcome your baby into the world. This can be a special keepsake to share with your child in the future.

**Attend Prenatal Classes:** Joining prenatal classes or support groups can provide opportunities to connect with other expectant mothers and share your experiences. Learning about pregnancy, childbirth, and parenting together can strengthen your bond with your baby.

**Create a Pregnancy Ritual:** Establish a special ritual or routine that you do regularly to connect with your baby. Whether it's a morning meditation, a nightly bedtime routine,a walk in the park, a walk through nature or a weekly prenatal yoga session, find a practice that resonates with you and your baby.

**Visualize Your Baby:** Take time to imagine what your baby might look like, how they'll move, and what their personality might be like. Visualizing your baby can help you feel more connected and excited about the journey ahead.

**Bond with Dad:** Encourage your partner to bond with the baby too. Attend prenatal appointments together, feel the baby's kicks, and talk about your hopes and dreams for your growing family. Sharing this experience can deepen your connection as a couple and as parents-to-be.

**Stay Healthy**: Taking care of yourself is one of the best ways to bond with your baby. Eat a balanced diet, stay hydrated, get regular exercise, and prioritize rest and relaxation. Your baby will benefit from your well-being, and you'll feel more connected knowing you're nurturing your baby from within.

Make sure to choose activities that resonate with you and your baby, and enjoy these special moments together.

# CHAPTER 5

# Third Trimester: Weeks 28-Birth

As you enter the third trimester, your baby's development enters its final stages, and your body undergoes significant changes in preparation for childbirth. Let's delve into the biological transformations and milestones that occur during this crucial period:

**Fetal Development:**
**Rapid Growth:** From week 28 until birth, your baby experiences a period of rapid growth and development. They continue to gain weight and size, with their body length increasing significantly.

**Organ Maturation:** During the third trimester, your baby's organs, including the lungs, brain, and digestive system, undergo further maturation and refinement to prepare for life outside the womb.

**Fetal Movement:** As your baby grows larger, you may notice a change in the pattern and intensity of their movements. While there may be less space for acrobatics, you should still feel regular movements and kicks, indicating that your baby is healthy and active.

**Positioning:** Towards the end of the third trimester, your baby typically settles into a head-down position in preparation for birth. This positioning allows for a smoother and more efficient delivery process.

**Physical Changes**:
**Maternal Weight Gain:** During the third trimester, you may experience a significant increase in weight as your baby continues to grow and develop. This weight gain is necessary to support the needs of your growing baby and prepare your body for childbirth.

**Braxton Hicks Contractions:** These "practice" contractions become more frequent and pronounced as you progress through the third trimester. While they may feel similar to true labor contractions, they are typically irregular and do not indicate the onset of labor.

**Pelvic Pressure and Discomfort:** As your baby descends lower into your pelvis in preparation for birth, you may experience increased pressure and discomfort in your pelvic area. This may be accompanied by back pain, pelvic pain, and difficulty walking or standing for long periods.

**Hormonal Changes:**
**Relaxin Production:** The hormone relaxin continues to be produced at higher levels during the third trimester. This hormone helps relax the

muscles and ligaments in your pelvis, allowing for easier passage of the baby during childbirth.

**Oxytocin Surges:** Towards the end of the third trimester, your body begins to produce higher levels of oxytocin, the "love hormone," which plays a crucial role in stimulating contractions and initiating labor.

**Emotional Changes:** Nesting Instinct: Many expectant mothers experience a strong urge to "nest" during the third trimester, characterized by a desire to prepare their home and environment for the arrival of the baby. This may involve activities such as organizing the nursery, washing baby clothes, and stocking up on supplies.

**Mixed Emotions:** As you approach the end of your pregnancy journey, you may experience a range of emotions, including excitement, anticipation, anxiety, and apprehension about childbirth and becoming a parent. It's important to acknowledge and address these feelings as they arise and seek support from your partner, family, and healthcare provider.

**Preparation for Birth:**
**Prenatal Check-ups:** During the third trimester, you'll continue to have regular prenatal check-ups with your healthcare provider to monitor your health and the baby's development. These appointments may include measurements of your belly,

ultrasounds, and discussions about your birth plan and preferences.

**Childbirth Education:** Consider attending childbirth education classes or workshops to learn about the stages of labor, pain management techniques, and newborn care. These classes can help you feel more prepared and confident as you approach childbirth.

**Final Preparations:** As your due date approaches, you'll need to make final preparations for childbirth, including packing your hospital bag with essential items,finalizing your birth plan, and arranging transportation to the hospital or birthing center.

**Signs of Labor:**
As you near the end of the third trimester, be on the lookout for signs of labor, including regular and increasingly intense contractions, the release of the mucus plug (indicating cervical changes), and the rupture of the amniotic sac (water breaking). If you experience any of these signs or have concerns about your symptoms, contact your healthcare provider for guidance.

# Preparing for Labor and Delivery

As your due date approaches, it's natural to feel a mix of excitement and anticipation about the arrival of your little one. Preparing for labor and delivery is an important part of ensuring a smooth and positive birth experience. Here's what you need to know:

**Educate Yourself:**
Take the time to learn about the labor and delivery process. Attend childbirth education classes or workshops where you can learn about the stages of labor, pain management techniques, breathing exercises, and relaxation techniques. Knowledge is power, and understanding what to expect can help alleviate anxiety and build confidence.

**Create a Birth Plan:**
Consider creating a birth plan outlining your preferences for labor and delivery. Your birth plan can include details such as where you'd like to give birth (hospital, birthing center, or home), who you'd like to have with you during labor, your preferences for pain management, and any special requests you have for the birth experience. Keep in mind that flexibility is key, and be prepared to adapt your plan as needed based on circumstances.

**Pack Your Hospital Bag:**
Pack a hospital bag with essential items you'll need for labor and delivery, as well as for your hospital stay afterward. Include items such as comfortable clothing, toiletries, snacks, water bottle, phone charger, birth plan, and any comfort items that will help you feel more at ease during labor. Don't forget to pack items for your baby, such as clothes, diapers, and blankets.

**Stay Active and Healthy:**
Maintain a healthy lifestyle during pregnancy by eating nutritious foods, staying hydrated, and getting regular exercise. Practice prenatal yoga, walking, swimming, or other gentle forms of exercise that can help prepare your body for labor and delivery. Staying active can also help reduce stress and promote relaxation.

**Practice Relaxation Techniques:**
Practice relaxation techniques such as deep breathing, visualization, and mindfulness meditation to help manage pain and reduce anxiety during labor. Practice these techniques regularly leading up to your due date so that they become second nature when the big day arrives. Remember to focus on staying calm and centered, and trust in your body's ability to give birth.

**Seek Support:**
Build a strong support network of family members, friends, and healthcare providers who will be there to support you during labor and delivery. Consider hiring a doula or birth coach to provide additional support and guidance throughout the birthing process. Having a supportive team by your side can make all the difference in having a positive birth experience.

**Trust Your Instincts:**
Above all, trust in yourself and your body's ability to give birth. Your body was made for this, and you are stronger and more capable than you realize. Listen to your instincts, communicate your needs and preferences to your healthcare provider, and surround yourself with positivity and encouragement as you prepare to welcome your baby into the world.

Preparing for labor and delivery is an exciting and empowering journey. By educating yourself, creating a birth plan, staying active and healthy, practicing relaxation techniques, seeking support, and trusting your instincts, you'll be well-prepared to embrace the miracle of childbirth with confidence and grace.

**Emergency Plan:** Discuss with your healthcare provider what to do in case of complications or emergencies during labor. Knowing the plan can provide peace of mind.

# Birth Plan Essentials

Creating a birth plan is a way for you to share your wishes and preferences with your healthcare team so they can help make your birth experience as comfortable and safe as possible.

Here are the essentials for a birth plan:

**Pain Management:**
This is about how you can manage any pain during labor. If you want medicine to help with pain, you can ask for it. If you prefer not to use medicine, there are other ways like breathing exercises, massage or getting in a warm bath to help you feel better.

**Labor Positions:**
You have different options for how you can sit or stand during labor. Some moms find it helpful to walk around, sit on a big ball, or even stand in the shower. You can choose what feels best for you.
Explain if you're open to trying different positions throughout labor or if you have specific preferences for the pushing stage.

**Delivery Environment:**
Think about what you'd like the room to be like when you're giving birth. You can ask for softer lights, play your favorite music, or bring comforting things from home. Also, you can decide who you want to be with you during labor, like your partner, family, or a friend.

**Medical Interventions:**
Sometimes doctors might need to help things along or assist with the birth. You can talk about whether you're okay with this or if you'd prefer them to wait and see if your body can do it on its own.
Also clarify your stance on interventions like induction of labor, augmentation (speeding up labor

with medication), or assisted delivery methods like forceps or vacuum extraction.

Discuss your preferences regarding episiotomy (surgical incision to widen the vaginal opening) and whether you prefer to avoid it if possible.

## Cord Clamping:

After the baby is born, there's a cord that connects them to you. You can decide if you want the cord to be cut right away or if you want to wait a little bit. Waiting can give your baby some extra blood that's good for them. (Delayed clamping allows more time for blood to transfer from the placenta to your baby, which can have health benefits).

## Skin-to-Skin Contact:

This means holding your baby against your skin right after they're born. It's a nice way for you two to get to know each other and helps your baby stay warm and calm and also helps with breastfeeding initiation.

Specify if you want uninterrupted skin-to-skin time for a certain period, such as the first hour after birth, known as the "golden hour."

## Breastfeeding:

If you plan to breastfeed, you can say so in your plan. You can also ask that your baby be put on your chest right away so they can start breastfeeding if you're both up for it.

State if you prefer not to have pacifiers, bottles, or formula given to your baby in the hospital to promote breastfeeding success.

**Newborn Procedures:**
Provide your preferences for routine newborn procedures, such as administering vitamin K injection, applying antibiotic eye ointment, and conducting newborn screening tests for conditions like hearing loss and metabolic disorders.
Consider whether you want these procedures performed immediately after birth or if you prefer to delay some of them to allow for bonding time with your baby.
(These are things the doctors and nurses do to check your baby and help them stay healthy. You can talk about when you want these things done and which ones are important to you).

Remember to discuss your birth plan with your healthcare provider and keep it flexible, as labor and delivery can be unpredictable.

# Anticipating Your Baby's Arrival

Anticipating the arrival of your baby can bring up a range of emotions, from excitement to nervousness. Discuss your feelings with your partner, family, and friends. It's okay to have mixed emotions, and sharing them can help ease any worries.

As your due date approaches, try to rest and take care of yourself. Get plenty of sleep, eat healthily, and engage in activities that help you relax, like reading, taking walks, or practicing prenatal yoga.

Remember, every pregnancy and birth experience is unique. Trust yourself and your body, and know that you're doing the best you can to prepare for your baby's arrival.

# The Golden Hour

The "Golden Hour" is a precious time immediately following the birth of your baby. Here's what it entails:

**Immediate Bonding:**
During the Golden Hour, you and your baby are encouraged to have uninterrupted skin-to-skin contact. This means holding your naked baby against your bare chest. This closeness helps regulate your baby's temperature, heartbeat, and breathing, while also promoting bonding and breastfeeding initiation.

**First Feed:**
The Golden Hour is an ideal time for your baby's first breastfeeding session. Babies are often alert and instinctively seek out the breast during this time. Breastfeeding during the Golden Hour can help establish a strong breastfeeding relationship and stimulate milk production.

**Emotional Connection:**
The Golden Hour provides an opportunity for you and your baby to connect emotionally. Your baby has just transitioned from the womb to the outside world, and being held close to you provides comfort and security during this significant transition.

**Promotes Health:**
Skin-to-skin contact during the Golden Hour has numerous health benefits for both you and your baby. It helps regulate your baby's body temperature, stabilizes their blood sugar levels, and promotes the release of hormones that aid in bonding and breastfeeding.

**Family Bonding:**
The Golden Hour isn't just for mom and baby. Partners and family members can also participate in this special time by offering support, encouragement, and skin-to-skin contact if desired.

**Delayed Procedures:**
Whenever possible, routine procedures such as weighing, measuring, and administering medications or vaccinations are delayed until after the Golden Hour. This allows you and your baby to fully experience this crucial bonding time without interruption.
Overall, the Golden Hour is a sacred time that marks the beginning of your journey as a parent.

It's a time to cherish, bond, and welcome your baby into the world with love and warmth.

# Necessary Tips on Shopping for Your Unborn Child

One essential aspect of preparation for the arrival of your child is shopping for your baby's needs. From adorable clothes to practical gear, navigating the world of baby shopping can feel overwhelming for first-time parents. However, with the right tips and guidance, you can shop smartly and confidently to ensure you have everything your little one needs when they arrive. Below are the necessary tips to help you make informed decisions and create a comfortable and safe environment for your growing family.

**Essentials First:** Start by getting the basics like clothes, diapers, a crib or bassinet, a car seat, and feeding supplies. These are the must-haves for when your baby arrives.

**Quality Over Quantity:** While it's tempting to buy everything cute you see, focus on quality items that are safe and durable. Look for reputable companies and read feedback from other parents.

**Baby Gear Checklist:** Create a checklist to keep track of what you need. This can include items like a stroller, baby carrier, diaper bag, baby bathtub, and baby monitor.

**Safety First:** When choosing baby gear, prioritize safety features. Make sure items like car seats, cribs, and high chairs meet safety standards and have no recalls.

**Clothing Sizes:** Babies grow quickly, so don't buy too many clothes in newborn sizes. Instead, get a mix of sizes ranging from newborn to 3-6 months to accommodate their growth.

**Consider Secondhand:** You can save money by buying gently used baby items like clothes, toys, and furniture. Just make sure to inspect them for safety and cleanliness.

**Breastfeeding and Bottle Feeding Supplies:** If you plan to breastfeed, consider getting a breast pump, nursing bras, and nipple cream. For bottle feeding, you'll need bottles, nipples, formula (if not breastfeeding exclusively), and a bottle sterilizer.

**Room Preparation:** Think about how you want to set up the nursery or sleeping area for your baby. Consider items like a changing table, dresser, and baby monitor to make caregiving easier.

**Baby Registry:** Consider creating a baby registry to share with family and friends. This can help them know what you need and can be a great way to get gifts for your baby shower.

**Budget Wisely:** Babies can be expensive, so set a budget and prioritize your purchases. Focus on the essentials first and consider spreading out purchases over time to manage costs.
Trust your instincts and choose items that feel right for you and your baby.

# Dora's Story

I realised I was pregnant in March 2019, prior to that I had been experiencing rapid weight gain, increased appetite and I usually felt tired in the mornings. I also had irregular periods back then, which has now been corrected medically, so I didn't even suspect I was pregnant since it was normal for me not to have my periods some months.

My husband and I were having a random conversations on a certain day and he joked about my weight gain, I immediately told him about how I had been feeling lately and he jokingly said we should take a pregnancy test.

I took the test using about three pregnancy strips and it came out positive. The moment I saw the positive sign on the pregnancy test, a rush of emotions overwhelmed me. Joy, excitement, and a hint of nervousness swirled together as I held the tiny stick in my trembling hands. I took a deep breath and called out to my husband, Tom.

From that moment on, Tom was my rock. He attended every doctor's appointment with me, holding my hand and asking thoughtful questions. When I was hit with morning sickness, he was there with ginger tea and crackers, rubbing my back and whispering words of comfort.

As my belly grew, so did our anticipation. Tom spent most of his free time preparing our home for the baby, he also read parenting books. Most nights, he would talk to our baby, his voice gentle and loving, his hands resting on my stomach.

There were tough days, of course. Days when I felt exhausted, my body aching from the strain of carrying our growing baby. On those days, I didn't fail to call my doctor to explain the exact way I was feeling, Tom was not left out, he would run me warm baths, massage my swollen feet, and remind me how amazing he thought I was.

As my due date approached, I found myself growing more anxious. Would I be a good mother? Would everything go smoothly?

Finally, the day arrived. My contractions started early in the morning, and Tom was by my side in an instant, timing them and helping me breathe through the pain. Labor was intense, more difficult than I had imagined. But through it all, Tom never left my side. He held my hand, whispered words of encouragement, and kept me focused on the end goal: meeting our baby.

And then, with one final push, our baby entered the world. This year our dear Ariel turned five and our love for her keeps growing. We currently have two more kids Jerry and Jimmy.

My advice to first time moms is this, take each day as it comes, know that you are not alone and always remember that motherhood is beautiful.

# Frequently Asked Questions and Answers.

Question 1: How can I manage morning sickness?

Answer: Eat small, frequent meals, stay hydrated, and avoid strong odors or foods that trigger nausea. Ginger and vitamin B6 pills may also be beneficial. For personalized advice, consult with your healthcare physician.

Question 2: Can I continue to drink coffee?

Answer: It's recommended to limit caffeine intake to 200 mg per day, which is about one 12-ounce cup of coffee. Excessive caffeine intake may be associated with an increased risk of miscarriage.

Question 3: What changes can I expect in the second trimester?

Answer: Many women experience relief from early pregnancy symptoms and feel more energetic. You may start to show a baby bump, and you'll likely feel the baby's movements (quickening) between 18-22 weeks.

Question 4: Is it safe to travel during the second trimester?

Answer: The second trimester is often considered the safest time to travel, as morning sickness has usually subsided and the risk of complications is lower. Before traveling, always consult with your healthcare physician.

Question 5: What prenatal tests are done in the second trimester?

Answer: Common tests include the anatomy scan (20-week ultrasound) to check for fetal development and abnormalities, and blood tests such as the glucose screening for gestational diabetes.

Question 6: How much weight should I gain during the second trimester?

Answer: Weight gain recommendations vary, but typically, women should aim to gain about 1-2 pounds per week. Total weight gain should align with your healthcare provider's guidelines based on your pre-pregnancy weight.

Question 7: Can I still sleep on my back?

Answer: It's recommended to start sleeping on your side, especially the left side, to improve blood flow to the baby. Use pillows to support your abdomen and back for comfort.

Question 8: How can I relieve back pain during pregnancy?

Answer: Maintain good posture, wear supportive shoes, avoid lifting heavy objects, and practice prenatal yoga or stretching exercises. A pregnancy support belt may also prove useful.

Question 9: What are common third trimester symptoms?

Answer: Common symptoms include shortness of breath, heartburn, swelling (edema) in the feet and ankles, Braxton Hicks contractions, and increased fatigue.

Question 10: When should I pack my hospital bag?

Answer: It's a good idea to have your hospital bag packed by 36 weeks. Include essentials like comfortable clothing, toiletries, baby clothes, and important documents.

Question 11: How can I tell if I'm experiencing preterm labor?

Answer: Signs of preterm labor include regular contractions, lower back pain, pelvic pressure, and changes in vaginal discharge. Contact your healthcare provider immediately ifyou experience these symptoms.

Question 12: What should I do if I think my water has broken?

Answer: If you suspect your water has broken, contact your healthcare provider or go to the hospital. It's important to get medical attention to prevent infection and assess labor progression.

Question 13: How often should I feel my baby move?

Answer: Fetal movements should be regular and consistent. You should feel at least 10 movements within two hours. Get in touch with your healthcare professional if you observe a decrease in movement.

Question 14: What is the difference between true labor and Braxton Hicks contractions?

Answer: True labor contractions are regular, increase in intensity, and become closer together over time. Braxton Hicks contractions are irregular, typically painless, and do not increase in severity or frequency.

Question 15: How important is prenatal nutrition?

Answer: Prenatal nutrition is crucial for your baby's growth and development. Focus on a balanced diet rich in fruits, vegetables, whole grains, lean proteins, and prenatal vitamins as recommended by your healthcare provider.

Question 16: What should I do if I experience bleeding during pregnancy?

Answer: Contact your healthcare provider immediately if you experience any bleeding during pregnancy. While some light spotting can be normal, bleeding can also indicate potential complications that need prompt attention.

# Chapter 6

# Labor and delivery

In this chapter, we'll explore the professional insights and essential tips to help you prepare for the momentous event of bringing your baby into the world. From the stages of labor to the role of healthcare providers, pain management options, and postpartum care, this is tailored to equip you with the knowledge and confidence needed for this transformative experience.

## Signs of labor

It's normal to be curious about the start of labor as your due date draws near. Understanding the signs of labor can help you recognize when it's time to contact your healthcare provider and prepare for the arrival of your baby. Here are the key signs to look out for:

**Contractions:**
Contractions are like waves of tightening and releasing in your belly. At first, they may feel like mild menstrual cramps, but as labor progresses, they become stronger, longer, and more regular.

Real labor contractions often begin in the lower back and extend to the abdomen's front. Usually, they approach at regular intervals and progressively move nearer to one another.

Timing contractions can help you determine if you're in labor. Use a stopwatch or smartphone app to measure the duration and frequency of your contractions.

## Water Breaking:

The amniotic sac, which surrounds and protects your baby in the womb, can rupture before or during labor. When this happen amniotic fluid may leak out in a trickle or gush.

If you suspect your water has broken, note the color and odor of the fluid. Clear or slightly pink fluid is normal, but if it's greenish or brownish, it could indicate a potential problem, and you should contact your healthcare provider immediately.

## Bloody Show:

The "bloody show" refers to the passage of a small amount of blood-tinged mucus from the cervix as it begins to soften and dilate in preparation for childbirth.

This discharge may appear pink, brown, or streaked with blood and is a sign that your body is getting ready for labor. It may occur days or hours before contractions begin.

**Back Pain:**

As your baby descends into the pelvis, you may experience increased pressure on your lower back, resulting in discomfort or pain.

Back pain during labor is often rhythmic and may come and go with contractions. Some women find relief by changing positions, using heat packs, or receiving massage from their partner or a doula.

**Pelvic Pressure:**

As your baby's head engages in the pelvis, you may feel increased pressure or heaviness in your pelvic area. This might make prolonged walking or standing uncomfortable. Some women describe a sensation of the baby "dropping" or settling lower into the pelvis, known as "lightening," as a sign that labor is approaching.

**Gastrointestinal Symptoms:**

Hormonal changes and the body's natural preparation for childbirth can lead to gastrointestinal symptoms like diarrhea, nausea, or vomiting in the hours leading up to labor.

These symptoms are thought to be caused by prostaglandins, hormones that help soften the cervix and stimulate contractions.

**Increased Discomfort:**

As labor approaches, you may notice an increase in overall discomfort, including abdominal cramping, pelvic pressure, and general unease.

This discomfort is often a sign that your body is gearing up for labor and is preparing to bring your baby into the world.

### Intuition:

Many women report a sense of knowing when labor is near, even before other signs become apparent. Trusting your intuition and paying attention to your body's signals can be a valuable indicator of impending labor.
If you have a strong feeling that labor is beginning, don't hesitate to contact your healthcare provider for guidance and reassurance.

# Coping Techniques for Labor Pain

As you prepare for the birth of your baby, it's natural to wonder how you'll cope with the discomforts of labor. Fortunately, there are many techniques you can use to manage and alleviate labor pain. Here are some easy-to-understand coping techniques:

### Breathing Techniques:

Deep breathing can help you stay calm and focused during contractions. Try inhaling through your nose and exhaling through your mouth while you take calm, deep breaths. You can also try rhythmic breathing, where you match your breaths to the rhythm of your contractions.

**Visualization**:
Visualization involves imagining a peaceful or comforting scene to distract yourself from the pain. Close your eyes and picture yourself in a serene place, like a beach or a garden. Focus on the sights, sounds, and sensations of your imaginary surroundings.

**Position Changes:**
Changing positions can help relieve pressure and discomfort during labor. Experiment with different positions, such as walking, rocking on a birth ball, or leaning on your partner for support. Gravity can also assist in moving your baby down the birth canal.

**Massage**:
Gentle massage can provide relief from tension and muscle pain. Ask your partner or labor support person to massage your lower back, shoulders, or feet during contractions. You can also use massage tools like a massage roller or tennis ball for self-massage.

**Warmth and Water:**
Warmth can help soothe labor pains. Take a warm shower or bath, or use a heating pad or hot water bottle on areas of discomfort. Some birthing centers offer hydrotherapy options, like laboring in a tub or whirlpool, which can provide significant pain relief.

**Counterpressure:**
Applying pressure to specific points on your body can help alleviate pain during contractions. You can use your hands, a partner's hands, or a massage tool to apply pressure to your lower back, hips, or thighs. Try out a variety of pressure points to see which suits you the best.

**Distraction:**
Keeping your mind occupied with distractions can help take your focus away from the pain. Listen to music, watch a movie, or engage in activities like reading or playing games during early labor. Having a supportive birth team to talk to and laugh with can also help distract you from discomfort.

**Guided Relaxation:**
Practicing relaxation techniques can help you stay calm and reduce tension during labor. Try listening to guided relaxation scripts or hypnobirthing tracks that lead you through progressive muscle relaxation and calming visualizations.

Remember, every woman's experience of labor pain is different, and what works for one may not work for another. Explore these coping techniques during your pregnancy to find out which ones resonate with you. And most importantly, trust in your body's ability to birth your baby and lean on your support team for encouragement and assistance throughout the process.

# Your Birth Team and Support System

As you prepare for the arrival of your baby, having a strong birth team and support system is crucial. These are the people who will support you emotionally, physically, and medically during labor and delivery. Here's a breakdown of who might be part of your birth team and how they can help:

**Spouse(Husband):**
Your spouse is often your main source of support. They can offer comfort, encouragement, and help you stay calm. They can also assist with tasks like timing contractions and communicating with the medical staff.

**Healthcare Provider:**
This can be an obstetrician (OB), midwife, or family doctor. They are responsible for monitoring your health and your baby's health during labor and delivery. They will guide you through the process and make medical decisions if necessary.

**Nurses:**
Nurses play a vital role in your care. They will monitor your progress, manage your pain, and provide support throughout labor. Nurses can also help with breastfeeding and newborn care after the birth.

**Doula**:
A doula is a trained professional who provides continuous physical and emotional support during labor and delivery. They can offer comfort measures, help with breathing techniques, and act as a liaison between you and the medical team.

**Family and Friends:**
You might choose to have close family members or friends with you during labor. They can offer additional support, encouragement, and help you feel more at ease. Make sure to discuss your wishes with them ahead of time.

**Childbirth Educator:**
A childbirth educator can provide you with information and techniques to prepare for labor. They often teach prenatal classes that cover topics like pain management, labor stages, and postpartum care. You and your spouse can benefit greatly from these classes.

**Lactation Consultant:**
If you plan to breastfeed, a lactation consultant can be a valuable part of your support team. They can help you and your baby with breastfeeding techniques and address any challenges that arise.

**Building Your Support System**
**Communication**: Discuss your birth plan and preferences with your birth team. Clear

communication helps everyone understand your wishes and work together effectively.

**Trust**: Choose people you trust and feel comfortable with. Your birth team should respect your decisions and support you through the process.

**Preparation:** Attend prenatal classes and meetings with your healthcare provider and doula. This will help you feel more prepared and confident about labor and delivery.

**Flexibility**: While it's great to have a plan, be prepared to adapt as needed. Labor can be unpredictable, and flexibility will help you stay calm and focused.

Having a supportive and knowledgeable birth team can make a significant difference in your labor and delivery experience. Surround yourself with people who understand your needs and can provide the care and encouragement you need as you welcome your baby into the world. Trust in your support system, and remember that you are not alone on this journey.

# Tiara's Story

Finding out I was pregnant was a moment I'll never forget. My husband, David, and I had been trying to have a baby for years. After two rounds of IVF, we were starting to lose hope. I remember sitting in the doctor's office, my heart pounding, waiting for the results. When the doctor finally said, "You're pregnant," I burst into tears. It felt like a dream come true.

David was over the moon when I told him. We hugged each other, both of us crying tears of joy and relief. It had been such a long journey, and now we were finally going to be parents.

The pregnancy itself was a mix of excitement and anxiety. Because of our history, every little twinge or symptom made me nervous. But David was my rock. He came to every appointment, held my hand, and reassured me that everything was going to be okay.

The first trimester was tough. I had terrible morning sickness and felt exhausted all the time. David took over most of the household chores and made sure I was eating well. He'd come home from work and immediately start cooking dinner or cleaning up, never complaining once.

As the pregnancy progressed, things started to get easier. We began to feel more confident and started planning for our baby's arrival. We spent weekends shopping for baby clothes and gear, always excited but still a bit cautious, not wanting to jinx anything.

As we got closer to the due date, the reality of becoming parents started to sink in. We took birthing classes together and read every book we could find on newborn care. David was always so involved, asking questions and making sure we were as prepared as possible.

Finally, the day arrived. My labour began at midnight and my husband was there to support me. When our baby finally arrived, we were both overwhelmed with emotion. Seeing our child for the first time, knowing how much we had gone through to get to this point, was indescribable.

Holding our baby in my arms, I felt an immense sense of gratitude. David had been my partner through every step of this journey, from the heartbreak of failed IVF attempts to the joy of finally becoming parents. His support and love had carried me through the toughest times.

Now, as we navigate the challenges and joys of parenthood together, I know we can handle anything. Our journey to get here wasn't easy, but it made us stronger. And every time I look at our baby, I'm reminded of how lucky we are to have each other and to finally have the family we dreamed of.

My advice to first time moms to be is this; Be patient with yourself and trust the process. Pregnancy, especially after IVF, can be filled with anxiety, but try to stay positive and enjoy each milestone. Maintain a healthy lifestyle, keep all your prenatal appointments, and lean on your partner and support system to help ease your worries.

# Questions And Answer Related this Chapter

Question 1: What are the stages of labor?

Answer: Labor is divided into three stages:
The first stage involves early labor, active labor, and the transition phase, where the cervix dilates from 0 to 10 centimeters.
The second stage is the pushing stage, where you deliver your baby.
The third stage is the delivery of the placenta.

Question 2: What are the signs that labor is starting?

Answer: Common signs of labor include regular contractions, water breaking, bloody show, lower back pain, pelvic pressure, gastrointestinal symptoms like diarrhea, increased discomfort, and a strong intuitive feeling.

Question 3: What are some natural ways to manage labor pain?

Answer: Natural pain management techniques include deep breathing, visualization, changing positions, massage, using warmth (like a warm bath or heating pad), applying counterpressure, and engaging in distractions like listening to music or watching a movie.

Question 4: Should I consider an epidural or other medical pain relief options?

Answer: Medical pain relief options, such as an epidural, are available if you find that natural methods aren't enough. Discuss your pain management preferences with your healthcare provider before labor begins.

Question 5: Who should be part of my birth team?

Answer: Your birth team may include your partner or spouse, a healthcare provider (obstetrician, midwife, or family doctor), nurses, a doula, close family and friends, a childbirth educator, and a lactation consultant.

Question 6: How can my partner support me during labor?

Answer: Your partner can support you by offering comfort and encouragement, helping with breathing techniques, providing massage, assisting with position changes, and being an advocate for your needs with the medical team.

Question 7: When should I go to the hospital or birthing center?

Answer: You should go to the hospital or birthing center when your contractions are 5 minutes apart, lasting 1 minute each, for at least 1 hour (the 5-1-1 rule), or if your water breaks. Always adhere to your healthcare provider's specific advice.

Question 8: What should I pack in my hospital bag?

Answer: Essentials include comfortable clothing, toiletries, important documents, a birth plan, baby clothes, a car seat for the baby, and personal comfort items like a pillow or music.

Question 9: What is a birth plan and do I need one?

Answer: A birth plan is a document that outlines your preferences for labor and delivery, such as pain management, labor positions, and who you want present. While not mandatory, it can help communicate your wishes to your healthcare team.

Question 10: What is an epidural and  does it work?

Answer: An epidural is a regional anesthesia that numbs the lower half of your body. It's administered through a catheter placed in the epidural space of your spine, providing pain relief during labor and delivery.

Question 11: Can I eat or drink during labor?

Answer: Policies vary, but generally, you may be allowed to have clear liquids like water, ice chips, and broth. Eating solid food is often discouraged, especially if there's a risk of needing general anesthesia.

Question 12: What is a cesarean section (C-section)?

Answer: A C-section is a surgical procedure to deliver a baby through an incision in the abdomen and uterus. It may be planned in advance or performed in an emergency if complications arise during labor.

Question 13: How long does labor usually last?

Answer: Labor duration varies, but for first-time mothers, active labor can last 12-24 hours. Subsequent labors are often shorter. The early labor phase can be longer, while active labor and pushing are typically more intense but shorter in duration.

Question 14: What is induction of labor and when is it necessary?

Answer: Induction of labor involves stimulating contractions before natural labor begins. It may be necessary for medical reasons such as overdue pregnancy, ruptured membranes without labor, or health concerns for the mother or baby.

Question 15: What is the role of a doula during labor?

Answer: A doula provides physical, emotional, and informational support during labor and delivery. Doulas do not perform medical tasks but help with comfort measures, advocacy, and continuous support.

Question 16: What are some common medical interventions during labor?

Answer: Common interventions include induction (using medications like Pitocin), artificial rupture of membranes (breaking the water), continuous fetal monitoring, and the use of forceps or vacuum extraction.

Question 17: What are the risks and benefits of an epidural?

Answer: Benefits of an epidural include significant pain relief and the ability to rest during labor. Risks may include low blood pressure, headache, and in rare cases, nerve damage or infection. Discuss with your provider to make an informed decision.

Q18: What should I expect during the delivery of the placenta?

Answer: After the baby is born, the placenta is delivered during the third stage of labor. Usually, this happens five to thirty minutes after birth. You may feel mild contractions, and your provider may help by gently pressing on your abdomen or asking you to push.

Question 19: What is skin-to-skin contact and why is it important?

Answer: Skin-to-skin contact involves placing the newborn directly on the mother's chest after birth. It promotes bonding, regulates the baby's temperature and heart rate, and supports breastfeeding initiation.

Question 20: How long will I stay in the hospital after delivery?

Answer: The typical hospital stay is 1-2 days for a vaginal delivery and 3-4 days for a C-section. However, this can vary based on your health, your baby's health, and any complications.

# Chapter 7

# Postpartum Period

Congratulations on the arrival of your baby! As you transition from pregnancy to parenthood, the postpartum period—often called the "fourth trimester"—brings its own unique set of experiences and adjustments. This crucial time begins right after childbirth and typically lasts for about six weeks. It's a period of profound physical recovery, emotional adjustment, and adaptation to your new role as a mother.

During the postpartum period, you'll experience changes in your body as it heals from childbirth, whether you had a vaginal delivery or a C-section. You may encounter physical symptoms such as bleeding, breast tenderness, and overall fatigue. Emotionally, this time can be a rollercoaster. Many new moms go through the "baby blues," characterized by mood swings and mild depression,while others may experience more severe postpartum depression, requiring additional support and intervention.

Caring for your newborn will also be a central focus, as you navigate feeding, sleep patterns, and bonding. Your baby will need frequent feedings, often every 2-3 hours, and will sleep in short stretches, which can be exhausting for you. Remember, taking care of yourself is just as important as taking care of your baby. Adequate rest, proper nutrition, and gentle physical activity when you're ready are essential for your recovery.

Your support system will play a vital role during this time. Don't hesitate to lean on your partner, family, and friends for help with household chores, cooking, and baby care. Regular check-ups with your healthcare provider will ensure that both you and your baby are healthy and thriving.

In this chapter, we'll explore the various aspects of the postpartum period, offering guidance and tips to help you navigate these first weeks with confidence and care. From physical recovery to emotional well-being, newborn care, and self-care strategies, we aim to provide you with the knowledge and reassurance you need to embrace this new chapter of motherhood.

## Recovery After Birth

Bringing a new life into the world is an incredible achievement, and your body needs time to recover from the journey of childbirth. Whether you had a vaginal delivery or a C-section, the postpartum period involves significant physical and emotional healing. Here's what you can expect and how you can support your recovery:

**Physical Recovery**
**1. Vaginal Birth Recovery:**
**Soreness and Swelling:**
It is common to experience soreness and swelling in the perineal area (the area between your vagina and anus). Ice packs and sitz baths can help reduce discomfort.

**Stitches:**
If you had an episiotomy or tear, you might have stitches. These usually dissolve on their own. Keep the area clean and dry to prevent infection.

**Bleeding:**
You will have vaginal bleeding and discharge, called lochia, for a few weeks. It will gradually change from bright red to pink, brown, and finally yellowish-white. Use sanitary pads and avoid tampons during this time.

**2. C-Section Recovery:**
**Incision Care:**
Your C-section incision will need special care. Keep the area clean and dry, and follow your doctor's instructions on how to care for it. Avoid heavy lifting and strenuous activities.

**Pain Management:**
You may experience pain at the incision site and general abdominal discomfort Your doctor will prescribe pain medication to help manage this.

### 3. Breast Changes:
**Engorgement:**
Your breasts may become engorged (swollen and tender) as they fill with milk. Frequent breastfeeding or pumping can help relieve this discomfort.
**Nipple Care:**
If you're breastfeeding, you might experience sore nipples. Use nipple cream and ensure your baby is latching correctly to minimize pain.

### Emotional Recovery
### 1. Baby Blues:
Many new moms experience mood swings, crying spells, and anxiety in the first two weeks after birth. This is known as the "baby blues" and is usually temporary. Rest, support from loved ones, and talking about your feelings can help.

### 2. Postpartum Depression:
If you feel intensely sad, hopeless, or overwhelmed for more than a few weeks, you might be experiencing postpartum depression. It is critical to seek assistance from your healthcare physician. Postpartum depression is treatable, and getting support early can make a big difference.

**Self-Care Tips**
**1. Rest:**
Sleep when your baby sleeps to help recover from childbirth. Newborns have irregular sleep patterns, so take naps whenever you can.

**2. Nutrition:**
Consume a diet high in fruits, vegetables, whole grains, lean meats, and balance. Staying hydrated is also crucial, especially if you are breastfeeding.

**3. Gentle Exercise:**
Start with gentle activities like walking when you feel ready. Your mood and energy levels can both be enhanced by exercise. Avoid strenuous exercise until you get the go-ahead from your healthcare provider.

**4. Accept Help:**
Don't hesitate to ask for and accept help from your partner, family, and friends. They can assist with household chores, cooking, and caring for the baby, giving you more time to rest and recover.

**Regular Check-ups**
**1. Postpartum Visit:**
Schedule a postpartum check-up with your healthcare provider around six weeks after birth. This visit is important to ensure you are healing well and to discuss any concerns you might have.

## 2. Newborn Check-ups:

Your baby will have several check-ups during the first year. These visits are essential to monitor your baby's growth and development and to address any health concerns.

Recovery after birth is a gradual process, and it's important to be kind to yourself during this time. Your body has gone through significant changes, and taking care of yourself is crucial. With proper care, support, and patience, you will gradually regain your strength and adjust to your new role as a mother.

# Newborn Care Basics

Welcoming your newborn home is an exciting and sometimes overwhelming experience, especially for first-time moms. Understanding the basics of newborn care can help you feel more confident and prepared. This section will guide you through the essential aspects of caring for your baby in those crucial first weeks and months.

## Feeding Your Newborn
### 1. Breastfeeding:
*Frequency:* Newborns typically need to eat every 2-3 hours, or about 8-12 times in 24 hours. Follow your baby's hunger cues, such as rooting, sucking on their hands, or crying.

*Latching:* Ensuring a good latch is key to successful breastfeeding. Your baby's mouth should cover both the nipple and part of the areola (the dark area around the nipple).

**Benefits**: Breast milk provides ideal nutrition, helps build your baby's immune system, and promotes bonding between you and your baby.

## 2. Formula Feeding:

*Choosing Formula:* If you choose to formula-feed, select a formula that meets your baby's nutritional needs. Your pediatrician can recommend a suitable option.

*Preparation*: Always follow the instructions on the formula packaging for proper mixing and storage. Use clean bottles and nipples.

*Feeding Schedule:* Like breastfed babies, formula-fed babies typically eat every 3-4 hours. Pay attention to hunger cues and adjust the amount as your baby grows.

## Sleep Patterns

### 1. Newborn Sleep:

*Sleep Duration*: Newborns sleep a lot—usually 16-18 hours a day. However, they wake frequently for feedings, typically every 2-4 hours.

*Safe Sleep Practices:* Always place your baby on their back to sleep, on a firm mattress in a crib or bassinet. Avoid soft bedding, pillows, and stuffed animals in the sleep area to reduce the risk of Sudden Infant Death Syndrome (SIDS).

### 2. Establishing a Routine:

***Day and Night:*** Help your baby distinguish between day and night by keeping daytime feedings and interactions lively and nighttime feedings calm and quiet.

***Consistent Schedule:*** Over time, try to establish a consistent feeding and sleeping schedule to help your baby develop a regular routine.

### Diapering

### 1. Diaper Types:

***Disposable Diapers:*** Convenient and widely available, but can be expensive and less environmentally friendly.

***Cloth Diapers:*** More cost-effective and eco-friendly but require more frequent washing and maintenance.

### 2. Diaper Changes:

***Frequency***: Change your baby's diaper every 2-3 hours, or whenever it's wet or soiled. Newborns may need up to 10-12 diaper changes a day.

***Preventing Diaper Rash:*** Keep the diaper area clean and dry. Use a barrier cream if needed, and allow your baby some diaper-free time each day to let their skin breathe.

**Bathing**
**1. Sponge Baths:**
Until the umbilical cord stump falls off (usually within the first two weeks), give your baby sponge baths instead of submersion baths.

*How to:* Use a soft washcloth and warm water to gently clean your baby's face, neck, hands, and diaper area.

**2. Tub Baths:**
Once the umbilical cord stump has healed, you can give your baby a tub bath 2-3 times a week.

*Safety Tips:* Use a small infant tub with a nonslip surface. Always support your baby's head and never leave them unattended during bath time.

**Umbilical Cord Care**
**1. Keeping It Clean:**
Maintain a dry, clean environment surrounding the stump of the umbilical chord. To minimize irritability, fold the diaper beneath the stump.
*Cleaning:* If the stump gets dirty, clean it with a cotton swab dipped in warm water and pat it dry.

**2. Monitoring:**
The stump should fall off within 1-2 weeks. Get in touch with your doctor if you observe any

infection-related symptoms, such as redness, swelling, or discharge.

**Baby's Health and Well-Being**
**1. Monitoring Development:**
Regular pediatrician visits are crucial to monitor your baby's growth and development. The doctor will check your baby's weight, length, and head circumference and ensure they are meeting developmental milestones.

**2. Immunizations:**
Vaccinations protect your baby from various diseases. Your pediatrician will provide a schedule of recommended immunizations.

**3. Recognizing Illness:**
Learn to recognize signs of illness, such as fever, unusual fussiness, poor feeding, or changes in bowel movements. If you have any concerns, contact your pediatrician.

**Bonding and Interaction**
**1. Skin-to-Skin Contact:**
Holding your infant skin-to-skin can assist regulate their body temperature, heart rate, and respiration. It also promotes bonding and breastfeeding.

**2. Communication:**
Talk, sing, and read to your baby often. Even though they may not understand the words, your

voice and facial expressions help them feel secure and start developing language skills.

### 3. Play and Stimulation:
Engage in gentle play and provide age-appropriate toys to stimulate your baby's senses and encourage their development. Simple activities like tummy time help strengthen their muscles and coordination.

Caring for a newborn can be challenging, but with patience and practice, you'll gain confidence in your abilities.

# Adjusting to Parenthood

Becoming a parent is one of life's most profound experiences, but it also comes with significant adjustments. As a first-time mom, it's natural to feel a mix of excitement and uncertainty as you navigate this new chapter in your life. Here are some key aspects to consider as you adjust to parenthood:

**Emotional Rollercoaster**
### 1. Hormonal Changes:
After giving birth, your body undergoes hormonal fluctuations that can affect your mood and emotions. It's common to experience mood swings, tearfulness, and feelings of overwhelm. Remember that these feelings are normal and will likely lessen over time.

**2. Bonding with Your Baby:**
Building a strong bond with your baby takes time and patience. Be gentle with yourself as you get to know your baby and learn to respond to their needs. Skin-to-skin contact, cuddling, and talking to your baby can help strengthen your connection.

**Sleep Deprivation**
**1. Newborn Sleep Patterns:**
Newborns have erratic sleep patterns and wake frequently to eat, usually every 2-3 hours. This can result in sleep deprivation for you as a new parent. Accepting help from your partner, family, or friends to share nighttime feedings can provide much-needed rest.

**2. Coping Strategies:**
While it's essential to prioritize your baby's needs, don't forget to take care of yourself too. Nap when your baby sleeps, even if it's just for short intervals. Creating a soothing bedtime routine for your baby can also help promote better sleep habits.

**Relationship Dynamics**
**1. Changes in Relationship Dynamics:**
The arrival of a baby can bring significant changes to your relationship with your partner. Adjusting to new roles and responsibilities can be challenging, but open communication and mutual support are key. Make time for each other, even if it's just a few minutes of quality time each day.

**Teamwork:**
Parenting is a team effort, and it's essential to work together with your partner as you navigate parenthood. Divide tasks and responsibilities based on each other's strengths and preferences, and be willing to adjust as needed.

**Self-Care**
**1. Prioritizing Self-Care:**
As a new parent, it's easy to prioritize your baby's needs above your own. However, taking care of yourself is crucial for your well-being and ability to care for your baby. Make time for activities that recharge you, whether it's reading a book, going for a walk, or enjoying a hot bath.

**Seeking Support:**
Don't hesitate to reach out for support from friends, family, or support groups for new parents. Sharing your experiences and seeking advice from others who have been through similar challenges can provide valuable reassurance and perspective.

**Adjusting Expectations**
**1. Embracing Imperfection:**
Parenthood is full of unexpected twists and turns, and it's okay if things don't always go according to plan. Embrace the imperfections and find joy in the small moments, even amidst the chaos.

**2. Flexibility is Key:**
Be willing to adapt and adjust your expectations as you learn and grow as a parent. What works for one family may not work for another, so trust your instincts and find what works best for you and your baby.

In conclusion, adjusting to parenthood is a journey filled with ups and downs, but with time, patience, and support, you will find your rhythm and confidence as a new parent. Remember that it's okay to seek help when you need it and to prioritize self-care amidst the demands of caring for your baby. Cherish the precious moments with your little one and trust in your ability to navigate this exciting new chapter in your life.

# Amanda's Story

Both of my pregnancies were truly enjoyable experiences for me. Aside from the common fatigue, irritability, and aches that come with carrying a baby, I found the process pleasant. Early on in my first pregnancy, I made a conscious decision to place my complete trust in God and my doctor. This decision played a crucial role in keeping me from overanalyzing or jumping to negative conclusions whenever I felt something was off. I focused on staying calm and breathing through any discomfort. This approach contributed significantly to my sense of peace and relaxation throughout both pregnancies. Toward the end, I even began to romanticize the experience, savoring the unique joy of nurturing the life growing inside me.

# Frequently Asked Questions About Postpartum

Question 1: How long does the postpartum period last?
Answer: The postpartum period, also known as the fourth trimester, typically lasts about six weeks after childbirth. However, physical and emotional recovery can take longer for some women.

Question 2: What physical changes can I expect postpartum?
Answer: Postpartum physical changes include vaginal bleeding (lochia), uterine contractions as it shrinks back to its normal size, breast engorgement, perineal discomfort, and potential swelling or soreness from a C-section incision.

Question 3: How can I manage postpartum bleeding?
Answer: Use sanitary pads to manage postpartum bleeding, which can last up to six weeks. To lessen the risk of infection, avoid using tampons at this time.

Question 4: When can I start exercising again after delivery?

Answer: You can generally start gentle exercises, like walking or pelvic floor exercises, a few days after a vaginal delivery if you feel up to it. For more intense workouts, wait until you get clearance from your healthcare provider, usually at your six-week postpartum check-up.

Question 5: How do I care for a C-section incision?
Answer: Keep the incision clean and dry. Follow your healthcare provider's instructions on wound care, and avoid heavy lifting and strenuous activities until you've healed. Keep an eye out for symptoms of infection, such as discharge, swelling, or redness.

Question 6: What is postpartum depression, and how do I know if I have it?
Answer: Postpartum depression is a serious condition characterized by persistent sadness, anxiety, irritability, and difficulty bonding with your baby. If these feelings last longer than two weeks or interfere with daily life, seek help from a healthcare provider.

Question 7: How can I manage postpartum pain and discomfort?
Answer: Pain management may include over-the-counter pain relievers like ibuprofen, using ice packs, sitz baths, and resting. Discuss any severe or persistent pain with your healthcare provider.

Question 8: When can I resume sexual activity postpartum?
Answer: It's generally safe to resume sexual activity once you've had your six-week postpartum check-up and have healed sufficiently. Ensure you feel comfortable and communicate with your partner about your readiness.

Question 9: What should I eat to aid postpartum recovery?
Answer: Consume a diet that is well-balanced and full of whole grains, fruits, vegetables, lean meats, and healthy fats. Staying hydrated and incorporating foods high in iron and fiber can also help with recovery.

Question 10: How can I boost my energy levels postpartum?
Answer: Get as much rest as possible, eat a nutritious diet, stay hydrated, and accept help from friends and family. Short naps and gentle exercise can also help boost your energy levels.

Question 11: How do I know if I have a postpartum infection?
Answer: Signs of infection include fever, chills, foul-smelling vaginal discharge, severe abdominal pain, or redness and swelling at the C-section site. Get in touch with your doctor if you encounter any of these signs.

Question 12: What is normal postpartum weight loss?

Answer: Initial postpartum weight loss includes the weight of the baby, placenta, and amniotic fluid, which is about 10-15 pounds. Gradual weight loss can continue over the next several months, but the timeline varies for each woman.

Question 13: How do I establish breastfeeding?

Answer: Start breastfeeding as soon as possible after birth, ideally within the first hour. Seek support from lactation consultants or breastfeeding support groups to help with latch and positioning issues.

Question 14: How can I manage postpartum hair loss?

Answer: Postpartum hair loss is common due to hormonal changes. It usually peaks around 3-6 months postpartum. Maintain a healthy diet, use gentle hair care products, and avoid excessive styling to minimize hair loss.

Question 15: When should I have my first postpartum check-up?

Answer: Your first postpartum check-up is typically scheduled around six weeks after delivery. This appointment allows your healthcare provider to check your recovery and address any concerns you may have.

Question 16: How can I bond with my baby postpartum?

Answer: Bonding can be fostered through skin-to-skin contact, breastfeeding, talking, singing, and spending time with your baby. Responding to your baby's cues and needs also helps strengthen your bond.

Question 17: What are the differences between postpartum depression and baby blues?
Answer: Baby blues are characterized by mood swings, tearfulness, and anxiety, typically occurring within the first two weeks postpartum. They usually resolve on their own. Postpartum depression is more severe and long-lasting, requiring medical attention.

Question 18: How can I manage postpartum hemorrhoids?
Answer: Use over-the-counter treatments, take sitz baths, eat a high-fiber diet, stay hydrated, and avoid straining during bowel movements. Consult your healthcare provider for persistent or severe cases.

Question 19: What should I do if breastfeeding is painful?
Answer: Pain during breastfeeding can be due to issues with latch or positioning. Seek advice from a lactation consultant, use nipple cream for soreness, and ensure your baby is latched correctly.

Question 20: How can my partner support me during the postpartum period?

Answer: Partners can provide support by helping with household chores, caring for the baby, offering emotional support, encouraging rest, and being understanding of the physical and emotional changes you're experiencing.

# Chapter 8

# Health and Wellness During Pregnancy

Congratulations on your pregnancy! This is a fascinating time of numerous changes, enthusiasm, and anticipation. As you embark on this journey, taking care of your health and wellness is more important than ever. The choices you make now can have a lasting impact on both your well-being and the growth and development of your baby.

In this chapter, we'll guide you through the essentials of staying healthy and feeling your best during pregnancy. We'll talk about the importance of eating a nutritious diet, finding safe and enjoyable ways to stay active, and the vital role of prenatal care. Ensuring you remain comfortable and happy throughout these nine months.

Whether it's your first pregnancy or you're adding to your family, this chapter is designed to provide you with the knowledge and reassurance you need to navigate this special time with confidence. By focusing on your health and wellness, you're giving your baby the best possible start in life. Let's dive in and explore how you can nurture yourself and your baby every step of the way.

# Nutrition and Exercise Guidelines

It is essential for you and your unborn child that you lead a healthy lifestyle during your pregnancy. Proper nutrition and regular exercise can help ensure a smoother pregnancy and a healthier baby. Whether you're a first-time mom or have been through pregnancy before, these guidelines can help you stay on track.

Nutrition Guidelines

1. Balanced Diet:
 Variety is Key: Aim to eat a variety of foods from all the food groups—fruits, vegetables, whole grains, proteins, and dairy. This ensures you get a range of essential nutrients.
Healthy Snacks: Choose nutrient-dense snacks like nuts, yogurt, fruits, and vegetables to keep your energy levels up throughout the day.

2. Essential Nutrients:
Folic Acid: Important for preventing neural tube defects. present in beans, fortified cereals, and leafy greens. Your doctor may also recommend a prenatal vitamin.
Iron: Helps prevent anemia and supports your baby's growth. Iron-fortified cereals, spinach, and lean meats are all good sources.

Calcium: Necessary for your baby's bone development. Good sources include leafy greens, dairy products, and fortified plant milks.
Protein: Essential for the growth of fetal tissue. Eat a diet rich in lean meats, chicken, fish, legumes, and tofu.
Omega-3 Fatty Acids: Vital for the Brain Development of Your Infant. Found in fish (like salmon), flaxseeds, and walnuts.

3. Hydration:
*Drink Plenty of Water: Aim for at least 8-10 glasses of water a day to stay hydrated, support digestion, and help with nutrient absorption.

4. Foods to Avoid:
Raw and Undercooked Foods: Avoid raw fish, undercooked meats, and eggs to reduce the risk of foodborne illnesses.
Certain Fish: Limit fish high in mercury, such as shark, swordfish, and king mackerel. Opt for safer options like salmon, tilapia, and shrimp.
Unpasteurized Products: Avoid unpasteurized milk and cheeses to prevent bacterial infections.
Caffeine and Alcohol: Limit caffeine intake and avoid alcohol to reduce risks to your baby's development.

Exercise Guidelines
1. Benefits of Exercise:
Improves Mood and Energy: Regular physical activity can boost your mood, increase your energy

levels, and reduce pregnancy-related discomforts like back pain.

Supports Healthy Weight Gain: Helps maintain a healthy weight during pregnancy.

Prepares Your Body for Labor: Strengthens muscles and improves endurance, which can be beneficial during labor and delivery.

2. Safe Exercises:

Walking: One easy and efficient approach to keep active is to walk. Set aside at least 30 minutes every day for this.

Swimming: Works your entire body without straining your joints.

Prenatal yoga: Promotes breathing exercises, relaxation, and flexibility.

Strength Training: Use light weights or resistance bands to keep muscles toned. Avoid heavy lifting.

3. Exercise Tips:

Listen to Your Body: Pay attention to how you feel and adjust your activities accordingly. Get medical attention and cease exercising if you have pain, lightheadedness, or dyspnea.

Maintain Hydration: Prior to, during, and following exercise, sip lots of water.

Avoid High-Risk Activities: Steer clear of activities with a high risk of falling or injury, such as contact sports, horseback riding, and skiing.

4. Consulting Your Healthcare Provider:

Medical Clearance: Before starting any new exercise routine, it's essential to get approval from your healthcare provider, especially if you have any pregnancy complications or concerns.

Adopting a balanced diet and staying active are key components of a healthy pregnancy. By focusing on nutritious foods and safe, enjoyable , you can support your well-being and give your baby the best possible start.

# Understanding Nutritional Needs During Pregnancy

Proper nutrition during pregnancy is essential for the health and development of your baby, as well as for maintaining your own well-being. Understanding what nutrients are most important and how to incorporate them into your diet can help ensure a healthy pregnancy.

Key Nutrients for Pregnancy

1. Folic Acid:
Importance: Folic acid is crucial for the prevention of neural tube defects, which affect the brain and spinal cord.
Sources: Leafy green vegetables (like spinach), citrus fruits, beans, and fortified cereals.

Recommendation: Most doctors recommend taking a prenatal vitamin that includes at least 400-800 micrograms of folic acid.

2. Iron:
Importance: Iron supports the increased blood volume during pregnancy and helps prevent anemia.
Sources: Lean meats, poultry, fish, beans, lentils, spinach, and iron-fortified cereals.
Recommendation: Aim for 27 milligrams of iron per day. Pair iron-rich foods with vitamin C (found in fruits like oranges and strawberries) to enhance absorption.

3. Calcium:
Importance: Calcium is essential for the development of your baby's bones and teeth.
Sources: Some of the sources include fortified plant-based milks, tofu, leafy greens, and dairy products (milk, cheese, and yogurt).
Recommendation: Aim for 1,000 milligrams of calcium per day. If you are under 18, you need 1,300 milligrams per day.

4. Protein:
Importance: Protein is vital for the growth of fetal tissue, including the brain, and also helps with the growth of your own breast and uterine tissue.
Sources: Lean meats, poultry, fish, eggs, beans, nuts, seeds, and tofu.

Recommendation: Aim for 71 grams of protein per day.

5. Omega-3 Fatty Acids:
Importance: Omega-3 fatty acids, particularly DHA, are important for your baby's brain and eye development.
Sources: Walnuts, chia seeds, flaxseeds, and fatty fish (such as salmon and sardines).
Recommendation: Aim for 200-300 milligrams of DHA daily.

Daily Nutritional Guidelines

1. Balanced Diet:
 Fruits and Vegetables: Include a variety of colorful fruits and vegetables to ensure you get a wide range of vitamins and minerals.
Whole Grains: Opt for whole grains like whole wheat bread, brown rice, oatmeal, and quinoa over refined grains.
Dairy or Alternatives: Include low-fat or fat-free dairy products or fortified plant-based alternatives for calcium and vitamin D.
Lean Proteins: Incorporate a variety of protein sources, such as lean meats, fish, eggs, beans, and nuts.

2. Hydration:
 Water: Aim to drink at least 8-10 glasses of water daily to stay hydrated, support digestion, and help with nutrient absorption.

Other Beverages: Limit caffeine and avoid sugary drinks and alcohol.

3. Portion Sizes:
Pay attention to your body's signals of hunger and fullness while eating in moderation. You don't need to "eat for two," but you will need slightly more calories, especially in the second and third trimesters.

Foods to Avoid

1. Certain Fish:
Steer clear of fish that are high in mercury, like swordfish, king mackerel, tilefish, and shark. Opt for safer fish like salmon, tilapia, and shrimp.

2. Raw and Undercooked Foods:
Avoid raw or undercooked fish, eggs, and meats to reduce the risk of foodborne illnesses.

3. Unpasteurized Products:
Stay away from unpasteurized milk and cheeses, which can carry harmful bacteria.

4. Caffeine and Alcohol:
Limit caffeine intake to less than 200 milligrams per day (about one 12-ounce cup of coffee) and avoid alcohol completely to prevent potential harm to your baby.

Understanding and meeting your nutritional needs during pregnancy is key to supporting your baby's development and maintaining your health.

# Essential Nutrients for Mom and Baby

During pregnancy, getting the right nutrients is vital for both you and your baby's health and development. Here's a simple guide to the essential nutrients you need and where to find them.

**Folic Acid**
**Why It's Important:**
Folic acid helps prevent neural tube defects, which affect your baby's brain and spinal cord.

**Where to Find It:**
- Leafy green vegetables (spinach, kale)
- Citrus fruits (oranges, lemons)
- Beans and lentils
- Fortified cereals

**Daily Amount:**
Aim for at least 400-800 micrograms (mcg) per day. Most prenatal vitamins contain this amount.

**Iron**
**Why It's Important:**
Iron contributes to increased blood volume during pregnancy and helps avoid anemia, which can induce weariness.

**Where to Find It:**
- Lean meats (beef, chicken)
- Fish
- Spinach and other leafy greens
- Iron-fortified cereals and breads

**Daily Amount:**
Aim for 27 milligrams (mg) per day. Combining iron-rich foods with vitamin C (found in fruits like oranges) can help improve absorption.

**Calcium**
**Why It's Important:**
Calcium is necessary for your baby's bone and tooth development.

**Where to Find It:**
- Dairy products (milk, cheese, yogurt)
- Fortified plant-based milks (almond milk, soy milk)
- Leafy greens (broccoli, kale)
- Tofu

**Daily Amount:**
Aim for 1,000 milligrams (mg) per day. If you are under 18, you need 1,300 mg per day.

**Protein**
**Why It's Important:**
Protein is essential for the formation of fetal tissue, including the brain, as well as the development of your own breast and uterine tissue.

**Where to Find It:**
- Lean meats (chicken, turkey)
- Fish and seafood
- Eggs
- Beans and lentils
- Nuts and seeds

**Daily Amount:**
Aim for about 71 grams (g) per day.

**Omega-3 Fatty Acids (DHA)**
**Why It's Important:**
DHA in particular is an essential component of omega-3 fatty acids for the development of your baby's brain and eyes.

**Where to Find It:**
- Fatty fish (salmon, sardines)
- Flaxseeds and chia seeds
- Walnuts
- Omega-3 fortified eggs

**Daily Amount:**
Aim for 200-300 milligrams (mg) of DHA per day.

**Vitamin D**
**Why It's Important:**
Vitamin D helps your body absorb calcium and
supports your baby's bone development.

**Where to Find It:**
- Sunlight exposure
- Fortified dairy products and plant-based milks
- Fatty fish (salmon, mackerel)
- Egg yolks

**Daily Amount:**
Aim for 600 International Units (IU) every day.

**Tips for Getting These Nutrients**
*Eat a Variety of Foods:* Include a mix of fruits, vegetables, whole grains, proteins, and dairy in your diet.

*Take Prenatal Vitamins:* They help fill any gaps in your nutrition and ensure you're getting essential nutrients.

*Keep Yourself Hydrated:* To promote general health and the absorption of nutrients, sip lots of water throughout the day.

*Consult Your Doctor:* Discuss your diet and any supplements with your healthcare provider to ensure you're meeting your nutritional needs.

Ensuring you get the right nutrients during pregnancy is crucial for your health and your baby's development. Focus on a balanced diet rich in essential nutrients, and take prenatal essential nutrients, and take prenatal vitamins as recommended by your doctor. By making mindful food choices, you can support a healthy pregnancy and give your baby a strong start in life.

# Foods to Emphasize and Avoid

Making smart food choices during pregnancy can help support your health and your baby's development. Here's a guide to the foods you should emphasize and those you should avoid.

**Foods to Emphasize**

*1. Fruits and Vegetables:*

*Why*: Packed with vitamins, minerals, and antioxidants that support both you and your baby's health.

*Examples:* Berries, oranges, leafy greens, carrots, broccoli.

*2. Whole Grains:*

*Why:* Provide essential nutrients like fiber, B vitamins, and minerals.

Examples include oatmeal, brown rice, quinoa, and whole wheat bread.

*3. Lean Proteins:*

*Why:* Important for your baby's growth and development.

*Examples*: Chicken, turkey, fish, beans, lentils, tofu.

4. *Dairy or Alternatives:*
*Why*: Good sources of calcium and vitamin D, essential for bone health.
*Examples*: Milk, yogurt, cheese, fortified plant-based milks.
5. *Healthy Fats:*

*Why*: Provide omega-3 fatty acids, important for brain and eye development.
*Examples:* Avocado, nuts, seeds, fatty fish (salmon, sardines).

## Foods to Avoid

### 1. High-Mercury Fish:
*Why*: High levels of mercury can harm your baby's developing nervous system.
*Examples*: Shark, swordfish, king mackerel, tilefish.

### 2. Raw or Undercooked Meat, Fish, and Eggs:
*Why*: Risk of foodborne illnesses like salmonella and listeria.
*Examples*: Sushi, raw oysters, rare steak, unpasteurized eggs.

### 3. Unpasteurized Dairy Products:
*Why*: Risk of bacterial infections like listeriosis.
*Examples:* Unpasteurized milk, soft cheeses (brie, feta, blue cheese).

### 4. Deli Meats and Processed Meats:
*Why*: Risk of listeria contamination.
*Examples*: Deli ham, hot dogs, bacon, salami.

5. **Excessive Caffeine:**
*Why*: High caffeine intake has been linked to low birth weight and miscarriage.
*Examples:* Avocado, nuts, seeds, fatty fish (salmon, sardines).

6. **Alcohol:**
*Why*: Can cause birth defects and developmental issues.
*Recommendation*: Avoid alcohol completely during pregnancy.

**Tips for Making Healthy Choices**
*Read Labels:* Look for whole, minimally processed foods with simple ingredients.
*Plan Balanced Meals:* Include a mix of protein, carbohydrates, and healthy fats in each meal.
*Stay Hydrated:* Drink enough of water throughout the day to maintain your general health and hydration.
Eat when you're hungry and pay heed to your body's signals of fullness and hunger.
*Consult Your Doctor:* If you have any questions or concerns about your diet, talk to your healthcare provider.
Emphasizing nutrient-rich foods and avoiding potentially harmful ones can help ensure a healthy pregnancy for you and your baby. By making informed food choices and prioritizing your health, you can lay the foundation for a positive pregnancy

experience and set the stage for your baby's future well-being.

# Creating Balanced Meals and Snacks

During pregnancy, it's essential to nourish your body with balanced meals and snacks to support your health and your baby's development. Here are some tips for creating nutritious and satisfying meals throughout the day:

Balanced Meals:
1. Include Protein:
Incorporate lean protein sources such as chicken, fish, tofu, beans, and lentils into your meals. Protein helps support your baby's growth and keeps you feeling full and satisfied.

2. Add Colorful Vegetables:
Fill half your dish with a variety of bright vegetables. Vegetables are rich in vitamins, minerals, and antioxidants essential for a healthy pregnancy.

3. Choose Whole Grains:
Choose whole grains such as brown rice, quinoa, whole wheat bread, and oatmeal. Whole grains provide fiber, B vitamins, and energy to keep you feeling fueled throughout the day.

4. Don't Forget Healthy Fats:
Include sources of healthy fats such as avocado, nuts, seeds, and olive oil in your meals. Healthy

fats are important for your baby's brain development and help absorb fat-soluble vitamins.

Balanced Snacks:
1. Pair Protein with Fiber:
Combine protein-rich foods like Greek yogurt, cheese, or nuts with high-fiber foods like fruits, vegetables, or whole grain crackers for a satisfying snack that stabilizes blood sugar levels.

2. Opt for Nutrient-Dense Options:
Choose snacks that provide a good balance of nutrients, such as hummus and veggies, apple slices with almond butter, or whole grain toast with avocado.

3. Keep Portions in Check:
Be mindful of portion sizes to avoid overeating. Aim for snacks that are around 150-200 calories and include a mix of protein, carbohydrates, and healthy fats.

4. Stay Hydrated:
Don't forget to drink plenty of water throughout the day, especially when snacking. Staying hydrated is essential for overall health and helps prevent dehydration, which can lead to fatigue and discomfort.
Planning Ahead:
1. Meal Prep:

Spend some time each week planning and preparing meals and snacks in advance. Having healthy options readily available can help you make better choices and avoid reaching for less nutritious options.

2. Listen to Your Body:
Pay attention to your hunger and fullness signals, and eat when you're hungry. Snack as needed throughout the day to maintain energy levels and prevent hunger-induced cravings.

3. Consult Your Healthcare Provider:
If you have any specific dietary concerns or questions, don't hesitate to speak with your healthcare provider or a registered dietitian. They can offer personalized guidance and support to help you meet your nutritional needs during pregnancy.

Creating balanced meals and snacks during pregnancy is essential for supporting your health and your baby's development. By focusing on nutrient-dense foods, portion control, and planning ahead, you can ensure you're getting the essential nutrients you need for a healthy pregnancy journey. Always pay attention to your health, stay hydrated, and consult your physician as necessary.

# Healthy Snack Ideas During Pregnancy

Healthy Snack Ideas During Pregnancy
Maintaining a healthy diet is important for both first-time and experienced pregnant women. Snacks can help keep your energy levels up and provide essential nutrients for you and your baby. Here are some healthy snack ideas:

**Fruits and Vegetables:**
1. Apple Slices with Almond Butter
- Provides fiber and healthy fats.
2. Carrot Sticks with Hummus
- A good source of beta-carotene and protein.
3. Banana with Peanut Butter
- Rich in potassium and healthy fats.
4. Mixed Berries
- Packed with antioxidants and vitamins.
5. Cucumber Slices with Tzatziki
- Refreshing and hydrating.

**Dairy and Alternatives:**
1. Greek Yogurt with Honey and Nuts
- High in protein and calcium.
2. Cottage Cheese with Pineapple Chunks
- A good mix of protein and vitamin C.
3. Cheese and Whole Grain Crackers
- Provides calcium and fiber.
4. Smoothie with Spinach, Banana, and Almond Milk
- A nutrient-dense drink with added greens.

5.  Frozen Yogurt Bites
- A cool and nutritious treat.

**Whole Grains and Nuts:**
1.  Whole Grain Toast with Avocado
- Rich in healthy fats and fiber.
2.  Oatmeal with Fresh Fruit
- Provides sustained energy and fiber.
3.  Trail mix: nuts, seeds, and dried fruit. a healthy combination of carbs, lipids, and proteins.
4.  Whole Grain Rice Cakes with Hummus
  - Light and crunchy with a protein boost.
5.  Granola Bars (Low Sugar)

**Convenient and nutritious on-the-go snack.**
**Protein-Rich Snacks:**
1.  Hard-Boiled Eggs
  - An excellent source of protein and essential nutrients.
2.  Edamame
  - High in protein and fiber.
3.  Turkey Roll-Ups with Avocado Slices
  - Lean protein with healthy fats.
4.  Roasted Chickpeas
  - Crunchy and high in protein and fiber.
5.  Lentil Salad Cups
  - Nutritious and protein-packed mini salads.

**Hydrating and Refreshing Snacks:**
1.  Watermelon Cubes

- Hydrating and low in calories.
2. Coconut Water
    - Hydrates and replenishes electrolytes.
3. Fruit-Infused Water
    - Adds flavor to water with vitamins.
4. Chilled Gazpacho Soup
    - A refreshing vegetable-based snack.
5. Frozen Grapes
    - Cool and sweet with hydration benefits.

**Tips for Healthy Snacking During Pregnancy:**

- Balance Nutrients: Aim for snacks that provide a mix of protein, healthy fats, and fiber to keep you satisfied and nourished.
- Portion Control: To prevent overindulging, monitor portion sizes.
- Stay hydrated by drinking plenty of water throughout the day.
- Plan Ahead: Prepare snacks in advance to have healthy options readily available.
- Listen to Your Body: Eat when you're hungry and choose snacks that make you feel good.

By incorporating these healthy snack ideas into your daily routine, you can support your pregnancy with balanced nutrition and maintain steady energy levels throughout the day.

# Staying Active Safely During Pregnancy

Maintaining an active lifestyle during pregnancy is beneficial for both first-time and experienced pregnant women. Regular exercise can help manage weight gain, reduce pregnancy discomforts, and prepare the body for labor and delivery. However, it is crucial to prioritize safety and choose appropriate activities. This section provides guidelines and tips for staying active safely during pregnancy.

**Benefits of Exercise During Pregnancy**

Participating in regular exercise while pregnant has several advantages.

- Improved Mood and Energy Levels: Exercise can boost endorphins, enhancing mood and energy.
- Better Sleep: Physical activity may help improve sleep quality.
- Reduced Pregnancy Discomforts: Regular movement can alleviate back pain, constipation, and swelling.
- Enhanced Fitness: Maintaining fitness levels can facilitate an easier labor and recovery postpartum.
- Weight Management: Exercise helps manage healthy weight gain during pregnancy.

**General Guidelines for Safe Exercise**

1. Consult Your Healthcare Provider:

Before beginning or continuing an exercise routine, consult with your healthcare provider to ensure it is safe for you and your baby.

2. Choose Low-Impact Activities:

Choose low-impact workouts to reduce your chance of getting hurt. Examples include walking, swimming, stationary cycling, and prenatal yoga.

3. Stay Hydrated:

To stay hydrated, sip on lots of water prior to, during, and following physical activity.

4. Avoid Overheating:

Exercise in a cool, well-ventilated environment, and avoid hot and humid conditions. Wear breathable clothing to prevent overheating.

5. Listen to Your Body:

Pay attention to your body's signals. Stop exercising and see your doctor if you feel any pain, lightheadedness, dyspnea, or other discomfort.

6. Warm-Up and Cool Down:

Always start with a gentle warm-up to prepare your muscles and end with a cool-down to relax your body.

**Exercises to Avoid During Pregnancy**
1. High-Impact Activities:
Avoid activities that involve jumping, running, or other high-impact movements that may increase the risk of injury.

2. Contact Sports:
Stay away from sports that carry a risk of abdominal trauma or falls, such as soccer, basketball, and skiing.

3. Exercises on Your Back:
After the first trimester, avoid exercises that require lying flat on your back, as they can reduce blood flow to the baby.

4. Hot Yoga and Hot Pilates:
Avoid exercises in hot environments to prevent overheating and dehydration.

**Tips for Staying Motivated**
1. Set Realistic Goals:
Establish achievable fitness goals that align with your pregnancy stage and fitness level.

2. Find a Workout Buddy:
Exercise with a friend or join a prenatal fitness class for motivation and support.

3. Keep a Routine:
Schedule regular exercise sessions to build consistency and make physical activity a part of your daily routine.

4. Track Your Progress:
Maintain a journal to track your exercise activities and how you feel. Celebrate milestones to stay motivated.

5. Focus on Enjoyment:
Choose activities you enjoy to make exercising fun and rewarding.

# Benefits of Exercise for Expecting Moms

Exercise during pregnancy offers a multitude of benefits for both the mother and the developing baby. Engaging in regular physical activity can help manage weight, improve mood, and prepare the body for labor and delivery. Here are the key benefits of exercise for expecting moms:

**1. Improved Mood and Mental Health**
- Reduced Stress and Anxiety:
Regular exercise helps to lower levels of stress hormones and increase endorphins, which can improve overall mood and reduce anxiety.

- Prevention of Depression:

Physical activity has been shown to reduce the risk of prenatal and postpartum depression by promoting emotional well-being and enhancing self-esteem.

## 2. Enhanced Physical Health

- Healthy Weight Management:

Exercise helps to maintain a healthy weight during pregnancy, which can prevent complications such as gestational diabetes and preeclampsia.

- Reduced Pregnancy Discomforts:

Regular physical activity can alleviate common pregnancy discomforts such as back pain constipation, bloating, and swelling.

- Improved Cardiovascular Health:

Exercise strengthens the heart and improves circulation, which benefits both the mother and the baby by ensuring adequate oxygen and nutrient delivery.

## 3. Preparation for Labor and Delivery

- Increased Strength and Endurance:

Building muscle strength and endurance through exercise can make labor easier and more manageable, as it requires significant physical effort.

- Better Pelvic Floor Health:

Strengthening the pelvic floor muscles through specific exercises can help support the weight of the growing baby and reduce the risk of urinary incontinence during and after pregnancy.

- Enhanced Flexibility and Balance:

Exercises that improve flexibility and balance can help the body adjust to the physical changes of pregnancy and prevent falls or injuries.

## 4. Faster Postpartum Recovery

- Improved Muscle Tone:

Maintaining muscle tone during pregnancy can aid in faster recovery after delivery and help regain pre-pregnancy fitness levels more quickly.

- Reduced Risk of Postpartum Complications:

Staying active during pregnancy can lower the risk of postpartum complications such as excessive weight retention and cardiovascular issues.

- Better Sleep:

Regular exercise promotes better sleep quality by helping to regulate sleep patterns and reduce pregnancy-related sleep disturbances.

## 5. Benefits for the Baby:

- Healthy Birth Weight:

Regular physical activity can help ensure a healthy birth weight for the baby, reducing the risk of complications associated with low or high birth weight.

- Improved Placental Function:

Exercise enhances blood flow to the placenta, improving its function and the delivery of oxygen and nutrients to the baby.

- Lower Risk of Chronic Diseases:

Babies born to mothers who exercise regularly during pregnancy may have a lower risk of developing chronic conditions

# Safe and Effective Pregnancy Exercises

It is very helpful for the mother and the unborn child to remain active during pregnancy. However, it is essential to choose exercises that are safe and effective, ensuring they support your changing body and the growing baby. This section outlines some of the best exercises for pregnant women, providing guidelines for each trimester.

**General Guidelines for Exercise During Pregnancy**

1. Consult Your Healthcare Provider:

Before starting any exercise routine, it's crucial to get approval from your healthcare provider to ensure it's safe for you and your baby.

2. Stay Hydrated:

Drink plenty of water to avoid dehydration before and after exercise.

3. Avoid Overheating:

Exercise in a cool, well-ventilated environment. Wear light, breathable clothing.

4. Listen to Your Body:

Pay attention to how you feel. If you experience discomfort, dizziness, shortness of breath, or pain, stop exercising and consult your healthcare provider.

5. Warm-Up and Cool Down:

Always begin with a gentle warm-up and end with a cool-down to prepare and relax your muscles.

# Recommended Exercises by Trimester

**First Trimester (Weeks 1-12)**
**Walking**:

- Benefits: Improves cardiovascular health without excessive strain.
- Guidelines: Aim for 30 minutes of brisk walking most days of the week.

**Swimming**:

- Benefits: Provides a full-body workout and relieves swelling and joint pain.
- Guidelines: Swim at a comfortable pace and avoid overly strenuous strokes.

**Prenatal Yoga**:

- Benefits: Increases balance, eases stress, and increases flexibility.
- Guidelines: Join a prenatal yoga class to learn poses that are safe and beneficial.

**Strength Training:**

- Benefits: Maintains muscle tone and strength.

- Guidelines: Use light weights or resistance bands. Focus on major muscle groups and avoid heavy lifting.

## Second Trimester (Weeks 13-26)
### Low-Impact Aerobics:
- Benefits: Boosts cardiovascular health without high impact on joints.
- Guidelines: Participate in low-impact aerobics classes designed for pregnancy.

### Stationary Cycling:
- Benefits: Offers a cardiovascular workout while being gentle on the joints.
- Guidelines: Use a stationary bike at a moderate intensity, ensuring the seat and handlebars are adjusted for comfort.

### Pelvic Floor Exercises (Kegels):
- Benefits: Strengthens the pelvic floor muscles, supporting the uterus, bladder, and bowels.
- Guidelines: Squeeze the muscles used to stop the flow of urine, hold for a few seconds, and then release. Do this several times a day, ten to fifteen times.

### Modified Strength Training:
- Benefits: Continues to build and maintain muscle strength.
- Guidelines: Focus on exercises that support the back, legs, and arms. Avoid lying flat on your back.

**Third Trimester (Weeks 27-40)**
**Walking**:

- Benefits: Maintains cardiovascular health and helps with energy levels.
- Guidelines: Continue walking regularly but adjust the pace and duration as needed for comfort.

**Swimming**:

- Benefits: Reduces swelling, improves circulation, and relieves back pain.
- Guidelines: Swim gently and avoid any strokes that cause discomfort.

**Prenatal Pilates:**

- Benefits: Strengthens the core, improves posture, and relieves back pain.
- Guidelines: Join a prenatal Pilates class to learn exercises that are safe and effective for the third trimester.

**Stretching**:

- Benefits: Maintains flexibility and reduces muscle tension.
- Guidelines: Focus on gentle stretches for the back, legs, and hips. Avoid any stretches that cause strain.

**Exercises to Avoid During Pregnancy**
- **High-Impact Activities:**

Avoid running, jumping, and other high-impact exercises that can strain your joints and ligaments.

- **Contact Sports:**
Steer clear of sports like soccer, basketball, and hockey that carry a risk of abdominal trauma or falls.
- **Hot Yoga and Hot Pilates:**
Avoid exercises in hot environments to prevent overheating and dehydration.

- **Exercises on Your Back:**
After the first trimester, avoid exercises that require lying flat on your back, as they can compress major blood vessels and reduce blood flow to the baby.

# Tips for Including Exercise in Your Daily Schedule

Staying active during pregnancy is essential for maintaining overall health and well-being, as well as supporting a healthy pregnancy and preparing your body for childbirth. However, finding ways to incorporate physical activity into your routine can sometimes feel challenging, especially as your body undergoes changes. Here are some practical tips to help you stay active and fit during pregnancy:

**1. Start Slowly and Gradually Increase Intensity**
Begin with low-impact activities such as walking, swimming, or prenatal yoga. Start with short sessions and gradually increase the duration and intensity as you feel comfortable

## 2. Schedule Regular Exercise Sessions

Make exercise a priority by putting it into your daily or weekly regimen. Aim for at least 30 minutes of moderate-intensity exercise most days of the week, if approved by your healthcare provider.

## 3. Choose Activities You Enjoy

Make sure you choose things that you look forward to and truly like. Whether it's dancing, hiking, or gardening, finding activities that bring you joy will make it easier to stay motivated and committed.

## 4. Involve Your Partner or Friends

Exercise with your partner, friends, or family members to make it a social activity. Not only does it provide motivation and support, but it also strengthens your relationships and creates memorable experiences.

## 5. Make It a Family Affair

If you have children, involve them in your exercise routine by going for family walks, bike rides, or playing active games together. It sets a positive example for them and promotes a healthy lifestyle for the whole family.

## 6. Incorporate Exercise into Daily Activities

Look for opportunities to incorporate physical activity into your daily routine, such as taking the stairs instead of the elevator, parking farther away from your destination, or doing household chores like vacuuming or gardening.

## 7. Try Prenatal Exercise Classes

Consider joining a prenatal exercise class tailored specifically for pregnant women. These classes are led by certified instructors who understand the unique needs and limitations of pregnant women and can provide safe and effective workouts.

## 8. Listen to Your Body

During exercising, pay attention to how your body feels. If you feel uncomfortable or have trouble breathing or dizzy, stop and relax. If you have any questions or concerns, always get in touch with your healthcare practitioner.

## 9. Stay Hydrated and Well-Nourished

Drink plenty of water before, during, and after exercise to stay hydrated. Give your body healthy nourishment to help muscle repair and energy production.

## 10. Be Flexible and Adapt

Be flexible with your exercise routine and adapt it to accommodate your changing needs and energy levels as your pregnancy progresses. Pay attention to your body and modify your routines as necessary.

**11. Set Realistic Goals and Celebrate Progress**
Set realistic fitness goals that align with your
pregnancy stage and listen to your body's cues. To
stay inspired and motivated, recognize and
appreciate your little accomplishments and
progress along the road.

**12. Prioritize Safety**
Always put safety first and pay attention to your
body's cues. Avoid activities that pose a risk of
falling or abdominal trauma, and consult with your
healthcare provider before starting any new
exercise program.

# Managing Pregnancy Discomforts

Pregnancy as we know, comes with its fair share of
discomforts. From nausea and fatigue to back pain
and swollen ankles, these discomforts are often
part of the package. However, there are various
strategies and remedies you can use to help
alleviate these symptoms and make your
pregnancy experience more comfortable. Here are
some tips for managing common pregnancy
discomforts:

**1. Nausea and Morning Sickness**
**How to manage it:**
**Eat Small, Frequent Meals:** Instead of large meals, opt for smaller, more frequent meals throughout the day to help prevent nausea.
**Stay Hydrated:** Sip on clear fluids like water, ginger tea, or lemon water to stay hydrated and ease nausea.
**Try Ginger:** Ginger has natural anti-nausea properties. Consider ginger tea, ginger candies, or ginger ale to help alleviate nausea.

**2. Fatigue**
**How to manage it:**
**Get Adequate Rest:** Pay attention to your body and make rest a priority. Take short naps during the day and aim for 7-9 hours of sleep at night.
**Stay Active:** While rest is essential, gentle exercise like walking or prenatal yoga can help boost energy levels.
**Delegate Tasks:** Don't be afraid to ask for help with household chores or other responsibilities to conserve energy.

**3. Back Pain**
**How to manage it:**
**Practice Good Posture:** Maintain proper posture while sitting, standing, and walking to alleviate strain on your back.
**Use Supportive Pillows:** Sleep with a pillow between your knees and under your abdomen to support your lower back.

**Try Prenatal Massage:** Consider scheduling a prenatal massage to help relieve tension and discomfort in your back muscles.

## 4. Swelling

**How to manage it:**

**Elevate Your Feet:** Spend time Avoid Trigger Foods: Spicy, acidic, beforeand fatty foods can trigger heartburn. Avoid these foods if they tend to aggravate your symptoms.

**Stay Hydrated:** Drinking plenty of water will help eliminate excess fluid from your system and minimize swelling.

**Avoid Standing or Sitting for Prolonged Periods:** Take regular breaks to move around and avoid sitting or standing in one position for too long.

## 5. Heartburn

**How to manage it:**

**Eat Smaller Meals:** Large meals can exacerbate heartburn. Consider consuming smaller yet more frequent meals daily.

**Avoid Trigger Foods:** Spicy, acidic, and fatty foods can trigger heartburn. Avoid these foods if they tend to aggravate your symptoms.

**Stay Upright After Eating:** Wait at least two to three hours after eating lying down to help prevent acid reflux.

## 6. Constipation

**How to manage it:**

**Eat High-Fiber Foods:** Include plenty of fiber-rich foods in your diet, such as fruits, vegetables, whole grains, and legumes, to promote regular bowel movements.

**Stay Hydrated:** Drink plenty of water throughout the day to help soften stools and ease constipation.

**Stay Active:** Gentle exercise, such as walking or swimming, can help stimulate bowel movements and relieve constipation.

## 7. Leg Cramps

**How to manage it:**

**Stay Hydrated:** Dehydration can contribute to leg cramps, so drink plenty of water throughout the day.

**Stretch Before Bed: Gentle** stretching exercises before bed, focusing on the calf muscles, can help prevent nighttime leg cramps.

**Maintain Proper Nutrition:** Ensure you're getting an adequate intake of calcium, magnesium, and potassium, as deficiencies in these nutrients can contribute to leg cramps.

## 8. Shortness of Breath

**How to manage it:**

**Practice Paced Breathing:** When you feel short of breath, focus on slow, deep breaths in through your nose and out through your mouth.

**Use Supportive Pillows:** Sleep with extra pillows to elevate your upper body and ease breathing discomfort.

**Avoid Overexertion:** Pace yourself and avoid activities that require excessive exertion to minimize shortness of breath.

# Self-Care Practices during pregnancy

Taking care of yourself during pregnancy is crucial for your physical and emotional well-being, as well as for the health of your baby. Practicing self-care can help alleviate stress, promote relaxation, and enhance your overall pregnancy experience. Here are some professional yet easy-to-comprehend self-care practices for first-time pregnant women and experienced moms alike:

### 1. Prioritize Rest and Sleep

Get Adequate Sleep: Aim for 7-9 hours of sleep per night and listen to your body's cues for additional rest during the day if needed.

**Establish a Bedtime Routine:** Create a peaceful sleep routine to inform your body that it is time to shut down. This may include activities like reading, gentle stretching, or taking a warm bath.

### 2. Practice Mindfulness and Relaxation Techniques

**Mindful Breathing:** Take a few moments each day to practice deep breathing exercises to promote relaxation and reduce stress.

**Prenatal Yoga or Meditation**: Consider joining a prenatal yoga class or practicing meditation to help calm your mind and connect with your body and baby.

### 3. Nurture Your Body with Healthy Nutrition

**Eat Nutrient-Dense Foods:** Focus on consuming a balanced diet rich in fruits, vegetables, whole grains,lean proteins, and healthy fats to support your own health and the development of your baby.
**Stay Hydrated:** Drink plenty of water throughout the day to stay hydrated and support optimal functioning of your body.

### 4. Stay Active with GenPregnancytle Exercise

Engage in Regular Physical Activity: Incorporate gentle exercises such as walking, swimming, or prenatal yoga into your routine to promote circulation, maintain strength and flexibility, and support overall well-being.

### 5. Connect with Your Support System

Seek Support: Reach out to your partner, family members, friends, or other expectant mothers for emotional support, advice, and encouragement throughout your pregnancy journey.
**Join a Support Group:** Consider joining a pregnancy support group or online community to connect with others who are experiencing similar challenges and joys.

**6. Take Time for Yourself**

Schedule "Me Time": Set aside regular time for activities that bring you joy and relaxation, whether it's reading a book, enjoying a hobby, or indulging in a prenatal massage.

**Delegate Responsibilities:** Don't hesitate to ask for help with household chores, childcare, or other responsibilities to free up time for self-care activities.

**7. Practice Body Positivity and Self-Compassion**

**Celebrate Your Body:** Embrace the changes happening to your body during pregnancy and focus on the incredible work it's doing to grow and nurture your baby.

**Practice Self-Compassion:** Be kind to yourself and recognize that it's okay to have moments of doubt, fear, or vulnerability. Allow yourself to prioritize your own needs and well-being.

# Nana's Story

My husband and I were eager to start a family, so I stopped taking birth control during our honeymoon in October, hoping to be pregnant by Christmas. However, I didn't get my period for several months afterward. Each negative pregnancy test increased my worry. Eventually, I visited a fertility specialist and was diagnosed with polycystic ovary syndrome (PCOS).

We began fertility treatments right away. I went through multiple rounds of Clomid and injectable medications to stimulate ovulation, but each cycle was long and difficult. After two failed IUIs, my ovaries released over 20 eggs on the third attempt, making IUI too risky. We decided to try IVF instead. I was optimistic, thinking I'd be pregnant within a month, but had to freeze all the embryos and wait for my body to be ready for transfer. The wait was agonizing. It seemed like everyone around me was getting pregnant effortlessly, which made me feel frustrated and envious.

After a month, we were cleared for the transfer. I finally got the positive pregnancy test I had longed for over a year. The first trimester was stressful, but I was fortunate to have a smooth pregnancy, a positive birth experience, and a beautiful baby girl. The following year, another round of IVF resulted in success. Unexpectedly, I conceived naturally with my third child.

My fertility journey was far from what I had imagined. Although I'm immensely grateful for my three healthy children, I'll never forget the emotional pain and struggle during that first year of trying to conceive.

# Chapter 9

# Partner's Role in Pregnancy

## My Journey as a Supportive Husband During Pregnancy

As I sit down to reflect on the past nine months, I can't help but feel an overwhelming sense of gratitude and joy for the journey my wife and I have embarked on together. From the moment we found out we were expecting, I made a promise to myself to be there for her every step of the way, and looking back, I am pleased to say that I kept my commitment.

The journey began with the news of our pregnancy, and as we shared in the excitement and anticipation of becoming parents, I knew that my role as a supportive husband had just begun. I made it my mission to educate myself about pregnancy and childbirth, devouring every book, article, and resource I could find to better understand what my wife was going through, and how I could best help her.

As the weeks turned into months, I witnessed firsthand the physical and emotional changes that pregnancy brought upon my wife. From the morning sickness and fatigue of the first trimester to the aches and pains of the third trimester, I stood by her side, offering comfort, encouragement, and unwavering support.

I made it a point to attend every prenatal appointment with her, holding her hand as we listened to the sound of our baby's heartbeat and marveling at the miracle of life growing inside her. I made sure she felt loved and cherished every step of the way, showering her with affection and reassurance, even on the days when she felt overwhelmed or uncertain.

As her body underwent the incredible transformation of pregnancy, I made sure to adapt and adjust to her changing needs. I took on more responsibilities around the house, helping with chores, cooking meals, and running errands so that she could rest and take care of herself and our growing baby.

As the due date drew near, I remained a steadfast source of strength and encouragement for my wife, reminding her of her incredible resilience and inner strength. And when the day finally arrived, I was by her side every step of the way, holding her hand through the highs and lows of labor and delivery, and rejoicing in the arrival of our beautiful baby.

Looking back on our journey together, I realize that being a supportive husband during pregnancy wasn't always easy, but it was without a doubt the most rewarding experience of my life. I learned that love knows no bounds when it comes to caring for the ones we hold dear, and I am forever grateful for the opportunity to be there for my wife and our precious baby every step of the way.

# Supporting Your Partner Through Pregnancy

Pregnancy is an exciting and transformative time, but it can also bring physical discomfort, emotional ups and downs, and numerous challenges. As a partner, your support is crucial in helping your pregnant partner navigate this journey with confidence and ease. Here are some ways you can offer meaningful support throughout the pregnancy:

**1. Educate Yourself**
Learn About Pregnancy: Take the time to read books, articles, and reputable online resources about pregnancy. Understanding the physical and emotional changes your partner is experiencing will help you empathize and provide better support.

**Attend Prenatal Classes:** Join your partner in prenatal classes. These classes often cover essential topics such as childbirth, breastfeeding, and newborn care, and they offer a chance to ask questions and prepare together.

## 2. Provide Emotional Support

Be a Good Listener: Listen to your partner's concerns, fears, and excitement. Validate her feelings and provide reassurance. Sometimes simply being present to listen can make a great difference.

**Encourage Open Communication:** Create a safe space for open and honest communication. Encourage your partner to share her thoughts and feelings, and be sure to express your own as well.

## 3. Be Involved in Prenatal Care

Attend Appointments: Whenever possible, accompany your partner to prenatal appointments. This shows your commitment and gives you both the opportunity to ask questions and stay informed about the pregnancy's progress.

**Support Health Choices:** Encourage your partner to follow her healthcare provider's advice regarding nutrition, exercise, and prenatal vitamins. Offer to join her in making healthy lifestyle changes.

## 4. Help with Physical Comfort

Assist with Chores: Pregnancy can be physically demanding. Help with household chores such as cooking, cleaning, and grocery shopping to alleviate some of the burden.

**Offer Comfort Measures:** Offer massages to ease back pain, run warm baths to help her relax, and ensure she has comfortable pillows and supports for sleeping.

## 5. Promote a Healthy Lifestyle

Encourage Healthy Eating: Help your partner maintain a balanced diet by preparing nutritious meals and snacks. Join her in eating healthily to show solidarity and support.

**Stay Active Together:** Engage in safe, pregnancy-friendly exercises such as walking, swimming, or prenatal yoga. Exercise can boost energy levels and improve mood for both of you.

## 6. Prepare for the Baby

Plan Together: Involve your partner in planning for the baby's arrival. Set up the nursery, shop for baby essentials, and discuss your parenting hopes and goals together.

**Create a Birth Plan:** Work together to create a birth plan that outlines your preferences for labor and delivery. Discuss pain management options, who will be present, and any other important details.

## 7. Take Care of Yourself

Maintain Your Well-being: Supporting your partner is easier when you're also taking care of your own physical and emotional health. Ensure you're getting enough rest, eating well, and finding ways to manage stress.

**Seek Support if Needed:** If you're feeling overwhelmed, consider joining a support group for expectant parents or seeking advice from friends and family who have been through the experience.

### 8. Be Patient and Adaptable

Adapt to Changes: Understand that your partner's needs and moods may fluctuate. Be patient and flexible, ready to offer support in whatever form it's needed at the moment.

**Celebrate Milestones:** Acknowledge and celebrate the milestones of pregnancy, such as hearing the baby's heartbeat, feeling the first kicks, and reaching each new trimester.

# Parenthood Planning Together

Parenthood is an incredible journey that requires teamwork, communication, and preparation. Planning for parenthood together not only strengthens your relationship but also ensures that both partners are aligned in their expectations, responsibilities, and goals. Whether you are first-time parents or expanding your family, thoughtful planning can make the transition smoother and more enjoyable. Here's how you can plan for parenthood together:

## 1. Open Communication

*Discuss Your Expectations:* Have open conversations about your hopes, dreams, and fears regarding parenthood. Discuss your roles and responsibilities, and how you envision sharing the workload.

*Set Goals Together:* Talk about your short-term and long-term goals as parents. This could include decisions about work-life balance, childcare, education, and parenting styles.

## 2. Financial Planning

Budget for Baby: Review your financial situation and create a budget that accounts for the additional expenses of having a baby, such as healthcare, diapers, clothing, and childcare.

*Save for the Future:* Consider starting a savings account for future expenses, including education and other significant milestones. Discuss life insurance, health insurance, and creating or updating your will to ensure your family is financially protected.

## 3. Preparing Your Home

*Create a Safe Environment:* Prepare your home for the arrival of your baby by setting up a nursery and ensuring that your living space is safe and baby-friendly. This includes baby-proofing areas and ensuring you have essential baby gear.

*Gather Essentials:* Make a list of baby essentials you'll need, such as a crib, stroller, car seat, and clothing. Plan your purchases together, considering what items are necessary and what you can borrow or buy second-hand.

## 4. Sharing Responsibilities

*Divide and Conquer:* Discuss and divide household and parenting responsibilities to ensure that both partners are contributing equally. This can help prevent feelings of overwhelm and ensure a balanced approach to parenting.

*Support Each Other.* Be prepared to support each other emotionally and physically. Understand that both partners will have their strengths and weaknesses, and work together to complement each other's efforts.

## 5.Education and Preparation

*Attend Classes Together:* Consider attending prenatal classes, childbirth education, and parenting workshops together. These classes provide valuable information and help both partners feel more prepared and confident.

*Read and Research:* Read books and articles about pregnancy, childbirth, and parenting. Share what you learn with each other and discuss how you can apply this knowledge to your own experience.

## 6. Building a Support Network

*Involve Family and Friends:* Don't hesitate to reach out to family and friends for support and advice. Having a strong support network can make a significant difference in your parenting journey.

*Join Support Groups:* Consider joining local or online support groups for expectant parents. These groups can provide valuable insights, shared experiences, and emotional support.

## 7. Planning for Work-Life Balance

*Discuss Maternity and Paternity Leave:* Plan for maternity and paternity leave, and discuss how you will manage work commitments during this period. Ensure that both partners have time to bond with the baby and support each other.

*Create a Flexible Plan:* Understand that plans may need to change as you navigate parenthood. Be flexible and willing to adjust your routines and expectations as needed.

## 8. Emotional Preparedness

*Acknowledge Changes:* Recognize that becoming parents will bring significant changes to your relationship and lifestyle. Be prepared to adapt and support each other through these changes.

*Practice Self-Care:* Encourage each other to take time for self-care and to maintain individual interests and hobbies. A healthy and happy parent is better equipped to care for their child.

Planning for parenthood together is an essential step in creating a strong, supportive foundation for your growing family. By communicating openly, sharing responsibilities, and preparing both financially and emotionally, you can navigate the challenges and joys of parenthood with confidence and unity. Remember that this journey is a partnership, and working together will help you build a loving and nurturing environment for your baby.

# Resources for Expecting Parents

Preparing for a new baby is an exciting journey, but it can also be overwhelming. Fortunately, there are many resources available to help expecting parents navigate this special time. Here's a guide to some of the most helpful resources you can turn to during pregnancy:

## 1. Books

- Pregnancy Guides: Books like "What to Expect When You're Expecting" by Heidi Murkoff and "The Mayo Clinic Guide to a Healthy Pregnancy" provide comprehensive information on every stage of pregnancy.

- Childbirth Preparation: Titles such as "Ina May's Guide to Childbirth" by Ina May Gaskin offer insights into labor and delivery.
- Parenting Books: Books like "The Happiest Baby on the Block" by Dr. Harvey Karp help new parents understand baby care and soothing techniques.

## 2. Online Resources

- Websites: Reputable websites like BabyCenter, The Bump, and WebMD offer articles, videos, and tools to track your pregnancy week by week.
- Forums and Communities: Online communities like those on Reddit (e.g., r/pregnant) or BabyCenter forums provide a space to ask questions, share experiences, and get support from other parents.

## 3. Prenatal Classes

- Childbirth Education Classes: These classes cover topics such as labor, delivery, pain management, and postpartum care. They are often available at hospitals or birthing centers.
- Breastfeeding Classes: Offered by hospitals, lactation consultants, or community centers, these classes teach breastfeeding techniques and tips.
- Newborn Care Classes: Learn about diapering, feeding, bathing, and other essential newborn care skills.

## 4. Healthcare Providers Obstetricians and Midwives: Regular appointments with your

obstetrician or midwife provide personalized medical advice and answers to your questions.

- Lactation Consultants: Certified lactation consultants can assist with breastfeeding concerns and provide in-person or virtual consultations.

## 5. Apps

- Pregnancy Trackers: Apps like Ovia, Glow Nurture, and What to Expect offer daily and weekly updates on your baby's development, along with tips and reminders.
- Contraction Timers: Apps like Full Term and Contraction Timer help track contractions when labor begins.

## 6. Support Groups

- Local Support Groups: Many communities offer support groups for expecting and new parents, often organized by hospitals, community centers, or parenting organizations.
- Online Support Groups: Virtual groups and social media communities allow you to connect with other expecting parents, share experiences, and receive emotional support.

## 7. Videos and Podcasts

- YouTube Channels: Channels like "Mama Natural" and "Sarah Lavonne" offer video content on pregnancy, childbirth, and parenting.
- Podcasts: Podcasts like "The Birth Hour" and "Pregnancy Confidential" provide

stories and advice from experts and other parents.

## 8. Government and Non-Profit Resources

- Healthy Start: A program offering support and resources for pregnant women, new mothers, and young children.
- WIC (Women, Infants, and Children): Provides nutritional support, breastfeeding counseling, and health care referrals for low-income pregnant women.

## 9. Books for Partners

- Books for Dads: Titles like "The Expectant Father" by Armin A. Brott and Jennifer Ash, and "Dude, You're Gonna Be a Dad!" by John Pfeiffer offer practical advice for fathers-to-be.
- Books for Partners: "We're Pregnant! The First Time Dad's Pregnancy Handbook" by Adrian Kulp helps partners understand how to support the pregnant person.

# Frequently Asked Questions by Husbands During Pregnancy

Question 1: How can I best support my wife during pregnancy?
Answer: Provide emotional support by listening and being patient, help with household chores, attend prenatal appointments, and educate yourself about pregnancy to understand what she's experiencing.

Question 2: What changes can I expect in my wife's mood and behavior?
Answer: Hormonal changes can cause mood swings, irritability, and emotional sensitivity. Be understanding, patient, and supportive. Encourage open communication about her feelings.

Question 3: How can I help my wife manage pregnancy symptoms like nausea and fatigue?
Answer: Encourage her to eat small, frequent meals, stay hydrated, and rest often. Help with meal preparation and household tasks to reduce her stress and workload.

Question 4: Should I attend prenatal appointments and classes?
Answer: Yes, attending appointments and classes shows your support, helps you stay informed, and allows you to be actively involved in the pregnancy journey. It also makes your relationship stronger.

Question 5: What should I do if my wife is experiencing severe pregnancy symptoms?
Answer: If she experiences severe symptoms like heavy bleeding, severe pain, or persistent vomiting, contact her healthcare provider immediately. It's important to address any potential complications promptly.

Question 6: How can I help prepare for the baby's arrival?

Answer: Participate in setting up the nursery, help with baby shopping, and assemble baby gear. Discuss parenting styles, birth plans, and childcare arrangements to ensure you're both prepared.

Question 7: What is a birth plan and should I be involved in creating it?
Answer: A birth plan outlines your wife's preferences for labor and delivery, including pain management and who she wants present. Your involvement is important to support her wishes and understand the plan.

Question 8: How can I support my wife during labor and delivery?
Answer: Be present, offer encouragement, help her with breathing and relaxation techniques, and be her advocate with the medical team. Your calm and supportive presence can make a significant difference.

Question 9: What should I pack in the hospital bag?
Answer: Pack essentials for both your wife and the baby, such as comfortable clothing, toiletries, baby clothes, and important documents. Include snacks, a phone charger, and items for your comfort as well.

Question 10: How can I bond with my baby before birth?
Answer: Talk to and gently touch your wife's belly, attend ultrasound appointments, and read books or

play music to the baby. These activities can help you feel connected to your unborn child.

Question 11: How can I manage my own stress and anxiety about becoming a parent?
Answer: Educate yourself about pregnancy and parenting, communicate openly with your wife, seek support from friends or support groups, and practice stress-relief techniques like exercise or meditation.

Question 12: What should I do if I feel left out during pregnancy?
Answer: Communicate your feelings with your wife and find ways to be involved, such as attending appointments, participating in baby preparations, and discussing your hopes and concerns about parenthood.

Question 13: How can I help my wife with breastfeeding after the baby is born?
Answer: Offer practical support by helping with positioning, bringing water or snacks, and encouraging her. Learn about breastfeeding challenges and how to assist, and support her emotionally.

Question 14: What should I know about postpartum recovery?
Answer: Understand that recovery can be physically and emotionally challenging. Help with baby care, household chores, and offer emotional

support. Encourage her to rest and follow her healthcare provider's advice.

Question 15: How can I be involved in nighttime feedings and diaper changes?
Answer: Take turns with nighttime feedings if your baby is bottle-fed, or handle diaper changes and soothing the baby back to sleep. Sharing these responsibilities helps your wife rest and strengthens your bond with the baby.

Question 16: If my wife is suffering from postpartum depression, what should I do?
Answer: Be supportive and understanding. Encourage her to seek help from a healthcare provider and offer to accompany her to appointments. Postpartum depression is so significant, it needs to be treated by a specialist.

Question 17: How can I maintain a strong relationship with my wife during pregnancy and after the baby is born?
Answer: Prioritize communication, spend quality time together, and continue to express love and appreciation. Make an effort to understand her needs and support each other through this transition.

# Chapter 10

# Recommended Journals and Websites

**Recommended Websites**

**1. BabyCenter (www.babycenter.com)**
BabyCenter offers a wealth of information on pregnancy, childbirth, and parenting. It features articles, videos, and interactive tools like due date calculators and pregnancy trackers.

**2. The Bump (www.thebump.com)**
The Bump provides week-by-week guides, expert advice, and community forums for expecting parents. It also offers a personalized app to track your pregnancy journey.

**3. What to Expect (www.whattoexpect.com)**
Based on the popular book, this website offers extensive resources, including articles, videos, and community forums. The What to Expect app also provides daily updates and tips.

**4. Mayo Clinic (www.mayoclinic.org/pregnancy)**
The Mayo Clinic's website offers reliable, evidence-based information on pregnancy health, symptoms, and medical advice. It is a trusted source for expecting parents.

**5. American Pregnancy Association (www.americanpregnancy.org)**
This non-profit organization provides information on a wide range of pregnancy topics, including nutrition, great resource for expecting parents.

**6. KellyMom (www.kellymom.com)**
KellyMom is a well-respected resource for breastfeeding and parenting information. It offers evidence-based articles and practical tips for new moms.

**7. La Leche League International (www.llli.org)**
La Leche League offers support and information on breastfeeding, including how-to guides, FAQs, and access to local support groups and meetings.

**8. Parents (www.parents.com)**
Parents.com covers a wide range of topics related to pregnancy, childbirth and parenting. It offers articles, expert advice, and community forums to connect with other parents.

These books and websites provide a wealth of information and support for expecting parents. Whether you're looking for detailed medical advice, practical tips, or emotional support, these resources will help you navigate the journey of pregnancy and early parenthood with confidence. Take the time to explore these recommendations, and choose the ones that best fit your needs and preferences. Remember, staying informed and prepared can make a significant difference in your pregnancy experience.classes

# Pregnancy and Parenting Classes

Pregnancy and parenting  are invaluable resources for expecting parents, offering education, support, and confidence as you prepare for the arrival of your baby. These classes cover a wide range of topics, from childbirth preparation to newborn care, ensuring that you feel ready for each stage of this exciting journey. Here's an overview of the types of classes available and what you can expect from them:

### 1. Childbirth Preparation Classes
Purpose: To prepare expecting parents for labor and delivery.

What You'll Learn:
- Stages of Labor: Understanding the phases of labor and what to expect during each stage.
- Pain Management: Techniques for managing pain, including breathing

exercises, relaxation techniques, and information on medical pain relief options.
- Labor Positions: Various positions that can help ease labor and promote comfort.
- Interventions: Information about common medical interventions such as epidurals, inductions, and cesarean sections.

- Birth Plans: How to create a birth plan that reflects your preferences and needs.

Benefits:
- Increased confidence and reduced anxiety about labor and delivery.
- Practical skills for managing labor pain and stress.
- A better understanding of your options and how to make informed decisions.

## 2. Breastfeeding Classes

Purpose: To educate parents about breastfeeding and provide practical tips and support.

What You'll Learn:
- Latching and Positioning: Techniques for helping your baby latch correctly and comfortably.
- Milk Supply: How to establish and maintain a healthy milk supply.
- Common Challenges: Solutions for common breastfeeding issues such as sore nipples, engorgement, and low milk supply.

- Pumping and Storage: Guidance on using breast pumps and storing breast milk safely.
- Weaning: Tips for transitioning your baby from breastfeeding to other forms of nutrition.

Benefits:
- Increased confidence in your ability to breastfeed successfully.
- Practical tips for overcoming common challenges.
- Support from lactation consultants and other breastfeeding parents.

### 3. Newborn Care Classes

Purpose: To prepare parents for caring for their newborns.

What You'll Learn:
- Diapering and Bathing: Basic techniques for changing diapers and bathing your baby.
- Feeding and Burping: How to feed your baby (breastfeeding, bottle-feeding) and techniques for burping.
- Sleep Patterns: Understanding newborn sleep patterns and tips for safe sleep.
- Soothing Techniques: Methods for calming a fussy baby, including swaddling, rocking, and using white noise.

- Health and Safety: Basic first aid, recognizing signs of illness, and baby-proofing your home.

Benefits:
- Practical skills for daily newborn care.
- Increased confidence in handling and caring for your baby.
- Knowledge of important health and safety practices.

## 4. Parenting Classes

Purpose: To provide guidance on parenting techniques and child development.

What You'll Learn:
- Developmental Milestones: Understanding physical, emotional, and cognitive milestones during the first year.

- Parenting Styles: Different approaches to parenting and finding the one that suits your family.

- Behavior Management: Techniques for managing common behavioral issues and fostering positive behaviors.

- Attachment and Bonding: Developing a close emotional bond with your child.

- Self-Care: Tips for maintaining your well-being while balancing parenting responsibilities.

Benefits:
- A deeper understanding of child development and behavior.
- Tools for positive parenting and effective communication with your child.
- Strategies for maintaining a healthy work-life balance.

## 5. Specialized Classes

Purpose: To address specific needs or interests of expecting parents.

Examples:
- Multiples Classes: Tailored for parents expecting twins or triplets, covering unique challenges and preparations.
- VBAC (Vaginal Birth After Cesarean) Classes: For parents who have had a previous cesarean and are planning a vaginal birth.
- Hypnobirthing Classes: Techniques for using self-hypnosis and deep relaxation during labor.

Benefits:
- Targeted information and support for your specific situation.

- Practical strategies for unique pregnancy and birth scenarios.
- Increased confidence and preparation for specialized circumstances.

# Finding Community Support

Navigating pregnancy and parenthood can be both exciting and overwhelming. Having a supportive community can make a world of difference during this transformative time. Here are some ways to find community support as you journey through pregnancy and into parenthood:

**1. Join Local Parenting Groups**

**Prenatal Classes**: Many hospitals and birthing centers offer prenatal classes where you can meet other expecting parents in your area. These classes provide an opportunity to learn together and form connections that can extend beyond pregnancy.

**Parenting Meetups:** Look for local parenting groups or meetups in your community. Websites like Meetup.com or Facebook groups often organize gatherings for expecting and new parents to connect, share experiences, and offer support.

**2. Online Communities**

**Social Media Groups:** Join online communities and forums for expecting and new parents. Platforms like Facebook, Reddit, and online parenting forums provide a space to ask questions, share concerns, and seek advice from others who are going through similar experiences.

**Pregnancy Apps**: Many pregnancy tracking apps offer community features where you can connect with other expectant parents who are at similar stages of pregnancy. These apps often include forums, groups, and chat features for sharing updates and support.

### 3. Attend Support Groups
**Breastfeeding Support Groups:** Look for local breastfeeding support groups or lactation consultant-led meetings. These groups provide a supportive environment for breastfeeding mothers to share tips, troubleshoot challenges, and offer encouragement.

**Postpartum Support Groups:** Postpartum support groups can be beneficial to new parents as they navigate the trials of early parenthood. These groups offer a safe space to discuss postpartum experiences, share resources, and receive emotional support.

### 4. Seek Out Parenting Classes and Workshops
**Parenting Classes:** Consider enrolling in parenting classes or workshops offered by local community centers, hospitals, or parenting organizations. These classes cover a range of topics, from newborn care to positive discipline techniques, and

provide an opportunity to connect with other parents.

**Baby and Me Classes:** Joining baby and me classes, such as mommy and me yoga or baby massage, can be a great way to bond with your baby while connecting with other parents. These classes often foster a sense of community and support among participants.

### 5.Utilize Online Resources
**Virtual Support Groups: If** in-person support groups are not accessible or convenient, consider joining virtual support groups or online communities. Many organizations offer online support forums, webinars, and chat groups for expecting and new parents.

**Bloggers and Influencers:** Follow parenting bloggers, influencers, and social media accounts that resonate with you. These individuals often share personal experiences, tips, and resources that can be helpful as you navigate pregnancy and parenthood.

### 6. Connect with Friends and Family
**Reach Out to Loved Ones:** Don't hesitate to lean on friends and family for support during pregnancy and early parenthood. Reach out to loved ones who have been through similar experiences or who can offer practical assistance and emotional encouragement.

**Create Your Support Network:** Build a network of trusted individuals who you can turn to for advice, assistance, and companionship throughout your pregnancy and parenting journey.

# Conclusion

As we come to the end of this journey together, we want to extend our heartfelt congratulations to you on your pregnancy. Whether you are the expecting mother or the supportive partner reading alongside her, we hope that this book has provided you with valuable information, guidance, and support as you prepare for the birth of your child.

Pregnancy is a miraculous and transformative experience, filled with anticipation, excitement, and perhaps a hint of apprehension. But through every milestone, every flutter of movement, and every moment of wonder, remember that you are not alone. You are part of a community of expectant parents who are embarking on this journey alongside you, each with their own hopes, fears, and dreams.

To the expecting mother: Trust in your body's ability to nurture and nourish new life. Embrace the changes, both physical and emotional, knowing that you are growing a precious gift within you. Allow yourself to lean on your partner for support, to seek guidance from healthcare providers, and to find solace in the shared experiences of other mothers-to-be.

To the supportive partner: Your presence, love, and support are invaluable during this time of transition. Take an active role in the pregnancy journey, from attending appointments and childbirth classes to offering comfort and encouragement when needed most. Your unwavering support will strengthen the bond between you and your partner as you embark on this new chapter together.

As you prepare to welcome your little one into the world, remember to cherish every moment, from the flutter of tiny kicks to the quiet moments of anticipation and reflection. Embrace the journey with open hearts and open minds, knowing that each step brings you closer to the miracle of new life.

May your days be filled with joy, your nights with peace, and your hearts with boundless love as you embark on this beautiful adventure of parenthood. From our hearts to yours, we wish you all the best on your journey ahead.

With love and warmest wishes,

Kayren K. Mariirk